WHAT IN THE WORLD IS IMMUNOTHERAPY FOR CANCER?

WHAT IN THE WORLD IS
IMMUNOTHERAPY FOR CANCER?

Dr. Austin Mardon · Sabika Sami · Laura Orsini · Hafsa Saleem · Maha Saleem
Lea Touliopoulos · Madeline Langier · Lydia Sochan · Khushi Shah
Katie Tulloch · Karanveer Kaushal · Kibrom Makaby · Madeleine Landell

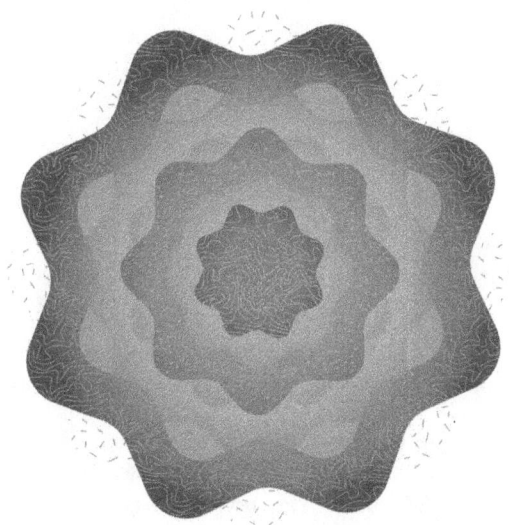

GM PRESS 2021

First Printing: 2021

Typeset, Cover Design & Illustrations by Coralie Larochelle

ISBN 978-1-77369-225-8

Golden Meteorite Press
103 11919 82 St NW
Edmonton, AB T5B 2W3
www.goldenmeteoritepress.com

CONTENTS

Sabika Sami

INTRODUCTION

Everyone has had their occasional colds and illnesses throughout their time on this Earth, like a stuffy nose, scratchy throat or inconvenient coughing. However, some of us are unfortunate, and we develop much more sinister and life-threatening diseases. Diseases that not only destroy the body but also destroy every other aspect of life. This is why it is critical in this modern-day and age that researchers find a solution to humanity's most prevalent disease; cancer. Unfortunately, in Canada, cancer is the leading cause of death at 30%, followed by heart disease (Ellison, 2009). Cancer treatment has always been dependent on plans to eliminate the tumour, such as surgery, chemotherapy and radiation therapy (Farkona, 2016). However, cancer immunotherapy is a treatment that has now only begun to be retrieved from the shadows. Unlike other cancer treatments, which target to eliminate the tumour, it still leaves a high chance of cancer developing again (Farkona, 2016). Cancer immunology is the treatment that grapples with the patient's immune system to fight back against cancer. Immunotherapeutic strategies include adoptive transfer, recombinant proteins and even cancer vaccines (Farkona, 2016). Throughout this book, cancer immunotherapy's challenges, trials, and tribulations will be discussed in detailed lengths.

THE CHALLENGE OF CANCER

It is estimated by the Canadian Cancer Society that, on average, 228 Canadians die from cancer every day (Lee, n.d.). The most common types of cancer, accounting for almost half of total cancer cases, are a cancer of the lung, breast, prostate, and colorectal (barring non-melanoma skin cancer). There are two main barriers identified by this chapter that hinder our ability to overcome cancer. Firstly, there are social factors that prevent life-saving cancer treatments from being accessed by marginalized populations. Secondly, there are scientific barriers that prevent us from accessing the means for a cure.

Across Canada, cancer diagnosis rates vary due to some areas being subject to increased exposure to carcinogenic materials. Furthermore, early detection is vital in increasing the likelihood of surviving a cancer diagnosis, but access to medical care is not equal among Canadian citizens. Both rates of exposure and access to resources are vital variables when analyzing the social determinants of health (Marmot, 2018). One study examining uterine cancer rates in Ontario found that marginalized communities tend to present more advanced cases and have a lower chance at survival on average (Helpman et al., 2020). Mammography screening is necessary for the early detection of breast cancer. The earlier the cancer is caught, the sooner intervention can begin, and the greater the likelihood survival becomes as a result. Immigrant and low-income women in the province of Ontario are less likely to receive this life-saving mammography screening, with South Asian women being the least likely to be screened (Vahabi et al., 2016). Socio-demographic factors have a life-altering impact on medical resource allocation, resulting in more minor resourced person devaluation.

Various factors contribute to one's likelihood of being diagnosed with and dying from cancer. The Canadian Cancer Society states that workplace exposure to hazardous materials and access to healthy foods are two predictive risk factors for cancer (n.d.). Of course, exposure to toxic materials is a job relegated to low-income and racialized persons. Having access to safe and healthy food is hardly equal among Canadian citizens. Several Indigenous populations in Ontario face unsafe drinking water advisories that have lasted for decades. The Human Rights Watch organization conducted a study in one such Indigenous community in which coliform and *E. coli*, uranium and trihalomethanes were discovered in the water (2020). Exposure to such toxic substances increases the rates of cancer in the area. Populations are told to boil their drinking water, but this is inconvenient, and many still bathe and wash their clothing in the contaminated water (ibid, 2020). These trends carry over to the American population as well. Racialized Americans are also privy to the social determinants of health. Alshareef et al. conducted a study analyzing the mortality rates of colorectal cancer patients. They found that Black and Indigenous persons were at a greater risk of dying from the disease than their white counterparts (2019). Various socio-demographic factors lead to racial disparities in the mortality risk of cancer patients.

Some argue that racialized persons are less likely to utilize cancer screening procedures which allow for earlier diagnosis (Shavers, 2002). There are also significant systemic environmental injustices that contribute to racialized persons having elevated health risks, including lead poisoning. The Flint, Michigan Water Crisis is an instance of environmental injustice that has hampered many people's health and livelihood (Campbell 2016). Residents of Flint, Michigan, were sourced with water that smelled and tasted foul. After many complaints were made, it was discovered that toxic lead was present in the water and other toxins that proved harmful to human health. The majority of the residents in Flint are African American and below the poverty line (Benz 2017). The Flint Water Crisis is part of a long-term trend of environmental racism, leading to increased health risks for marginalized communities. Also, due to environmental racism, Boynton, Michigan, is experiencing an elevated cancer diagnosis and cancer-related deaths (Benz, 2017). These consistently high rates of cancer for residents in Boynton are attributable to benzene. Benzene is a toxic substance that is known to be carcinogenic. Of course, Boynton is over 90% Black in its population, underscoring the trend of racial disparities in health outcomes (Benz, 2017).

Along with environmental racism, access to safe and healthy food also contributes to disparities in cancer diagnosis and cancer mortality rates. Food deserts are areas that do not have reliable access to healthy foods typically sourced from supermarkets. Due to this lack of access, residents of food deserts tend to have poorer health outcomes (Fong et al., 2021). Contrary to popular belief, Ivers found that food deserts are associated with poor health outcomes over and above simple obesity. One's location negatively impacted mental health in a food desert and fetal micronutrient deficiencies and toxin exposure from improperly prepared foods (Ivers, 2015). Income and geographic location are determinative of one's ability to access safe and healthy foods. The lack of financial accessibility to healthy foods in more impoverished areas leads to an obesogenic population (Nash, 2015). Obesity-related illnesses are plentiful, cancer being one of them.

Understanding the social determinants of health is imperative in guiding public policy goals for mitigating the severity and number of cancer cases in a given population. Individual scientists and learning institutions should also be mindful of the socio-demographic features which contribute to racial, economic and gender inequalities in health outcomes. The challenge of cancer is not merely a scientific one. Cancer is enmeshed in social circumstances which are hardly neutral to all persons. The subjectivity of a patient's identity can impact how they are treated by medical professionals regardless of whether there is a scientific solution to what ails them. The barriers to solving cancer are varied and complex, requiring an interdisciplinary approach to be taken up by all those in the medical and scientific research field.

In the spirit of taking a multidisciplinary approach and looking at the impacts of race on health outcomes, we can now look at the effects of gender on health disparities. Women are treated differently from their male counterparts in all sectors of society based on their gender, but this is particularly problematic when medical professionals treat women. Unsubstantiated notions of the fragility of the female form have long been a problem in the medical field. For example, studies have shown that when a woman complains of pain, she is more likely to be dismissed than male patients (Chen et al., 2008). This could have severe consequences on women's health, suffering from painful and potentially deadly health conditions, which medical professionals dismiss as exaggerating their symptoms despite their pain.

There are also some unfortunate, more systemic problems that prevent women from receiving adequate medical care. Women are often under-represented in medical studies, which leads to non-gender-transferrable treatments being developed for men but not for women. The male body is thought to be the default for medical research, but women are considered to have gender-specific traits which diverge from the male norm. So women are chronically understudied and underserved by the medical community (Holdcroft et al., 2007). Doctors are often less familiar with the symptoms presented by women suffering from heart attacks than men suffering from heart attacks. This results in delays in diagnosis that impact female sufferers' health prospects of heart attacks (Maserejian et al., 2009). This establishes that biases in medical research and medical practitioners can lead to poorer health outcomes for women. This is yet another social barrier that ought to be transcended if we meet the challenge of cancer equitably and does not further underserved, marginalized populations. Of course, this is not to say the medical professionals are a particularly racist or sexist group. Instead, the system is flawed.

Immunotherapy treatments for cancer are also impacted by social factors, which hamper our ability to treat all cancer patients reasonably regardless of race and gender. In a peer-reviewed study, Waqar et al. found that African American patients were less likely to receive immunotherapy treatment for metastatic melanoma in the United States. This finding is made even more significant given that Waqar et al. also found that those who did receive immunotherapy treatments for metastatic melanoma were more likely to recover than those who received no such treatment (2019). This study also found inequalities in access to immunotherapy treatments based on the economic status of the patients involved. The utilization of immunotherapy to treat metastatic melanoma is increasing, but it is not growing equitably. As a promising new treatment for cancer, immunotherapy treatment ought to be equalized so that the lives of cancer patients are not devalued on account of race and economic status. Diminishing racial disparities in immunotherapy ought to be a public health priority.

Verma et al. also studied racial disparities in immunotherapy treatments for lung cancer. They found that even when controlling for medicare, Medicaid and insurance differences, African Americans were still less likely to receive immunotherapy treatments for cancer (Verma et al., 2019). Excluding marginalized persons from receiving life-saving treatment, though it is likely caused by unconscious bias, needs to be consciously and decisively undermined by medical professionals and progressive public health legislation.

As one of the leading causes of death in the United States and Canada, early screening practices are imperative for preventing unnecessary deaths due to cancer. However, due to the Covid-19 pandemic, many appointments for cancer screening have been delayed if not cancelled outright (Patt et al. 2020). A delayed cancer diagnosis can lead to increased mortality, as cancers that would have been caught in the early stages of their development have now progressed and become more life-threatening. Those just now noticing signs of cancer may also have their screenings delayed for medical workers to drudge through the backlog of cases postponed by the Covid-19 pandemic (Patt et al. 2020). Many Canadians and Americans alike have lost their jobs or lost wages due to the Covid-19 pandemic. Some individuals may no longer have insurance and are now unable to receive life-saving cancer screenings; others may simply be too busy taking care of ill loved ones to take the time to screen for cancer.

As was mentioned briefly earlier, the problem of cancer can be broken down into two major categories: firstly, the social determinants of health create barriers in accessing life-saving medical intervention for cancer. Secondly, there are scientific advancements yet to be made in the creation and implementation of treatment methodologies. Therefore, the scientific community is tasked with developing such technological solutions equitably; this is no easy feat. Chakraborty and Rahman list seven key barriers to overcoming cancer (Chakraborty & Rahman, 2012). These problems include:

1. 'Targeting cancer stem cells is difficult'
2. 'Drug resistance properties of cancer stem cells make them immune to anticancer drugs'
3. 'Lack of cancer epigenetic profiling and specificity of existing epi-drugs'
4. 'Problems associated with cancer diagnosis make it difficult to treat'
5. 'Unavailability of effective biomarkers for cancer diagnosis and prognosis
6. 'Limitations of conventional chemotherapeutic agents'
7. 'Metastasis poses a huge problem in cancer treatment' (Chakraborty & Rahman, 2012).

1. 'Targeting cancer stem cells (CSCs) is difficult.'

It is primarily believed that cancer cells originate from stem cells. Many cancer treatments can eliminate the bulk of a cancerous tumour, but rooting out the cancer stem cell (CSC) has proven to be more difficult. This is problematic because the cancer stem cell can multiply after the treatments stop if left in the host. As a result, much about CSCs remains to be discovered. For example, the nature of the CSC mutation process is still very mysterious to cancer researchers. For this reason, Chakraborty and Rahman suggest that further research be conducted to discover the biology of CSCs (Chakraborty & Rahman, 2012).

2. 'Drug resistance properties of cancer stem cells make them immune to anticancer drugs'

Like most biological organisms, cancer cells fight to protect themselves from dangers, such as anticancer drugs developed to undermine them. For instance, chemotherapeutic medicine treatments target the rapid cell division, which creates the tumour, but CSCs are not the more populated cells in the tumour. CSC's divide less rapidly and are less likely to be targeted by treatments that target the hallmark rapid cell division (Chakraborty & Rahman, 2012).

3. 'Lack of cancer epigenetic profiling and specificity of existing epi-drugs.'

In this section, Chakraborty and Rahman discuss how the DMNT enzyme guides tumour suppression, and so the enzyme has become an obvious target for cancer researchers. The problem with the utilization of DMNT blockers in cancer treatment lies in its lack of specificity. This sort of treatment could lead to side effects such as the reactivation of genes that would normally be silenced post-puberty. According to Chakraborty and Rahman, the heritable changes in gene expression (epigenetics) are often studied in cancer research. Still, cancer researchers must focus on creating an epigenetic DMNT blocker that poses a greater degree of specificity (Chakraborty & Rahman, 2012).

4. 'Problems associated with cancer diagnosis make it difficult to treat.'

Along with the socio-demographic and economic barrier that prevents marginalized communities from receiving timely cancer treatment, disease-specific characteristics make identifying and treating cancer more difficult. For instance, some varieties of cancer may be asymptomatic, such that a person may have no way of knowing that cancerous tissue is growing within their body. For example, prostate cancer does not present any warning signs in the early stages of its appearance. Pancreatic cancer is also challenging to identify, as symptoms vary between patients (Chakraborty & Rahman, 2012).

5. 'Unavailability of effective biomarkers for cancer diagnosis and prognosis.'

Reliable, predictive biomarkers have yet to be discovered for cancer. The discovery of such biomarkers would allow for a more remarkable ability to comprehend the disease progression of cancer and assist in early detection (Chakraborty & Rahman, 2012).

6. 'Limitations of conventional chemotherapeutic agents

Chemotherapy is toxic. It destroys cancerous and non-cancerous cells, which results in hair loss typically seen in patients undergoing chemotherapy (Chakraborty & Rahman, 2012).

7. 'Metastasis poses a huge problem in cancer treatment.'

Cancer cells begin to grow in one specific area of the body, but they also acquire the capacity to colonize other areas of the body, creating secondary cancer sites. Thus, cancer cells can spread in multiple ways, one of which is through the bloodstream. When cancer metastasizes, it makes these secondary sites which require additional medical intervention.

The problem of cancer is not merely one problem; instead, there is a litany of the issues contributing to our inability to cure cancer, making the pursuit of most cancer researchers, by and large, an upward battle. This is not to say that the end of cancer is not in sight, however. With the progress of innovative new cancer treatment procedures (such as utilizing the immune system in immunotherapy), there is light at the end of the tunnel. As we broach the future of cancer, we must keep in mind the social factors that could impede our ability to diffuse the benefits of a hypothetical cure to cancer throughout all persons regardless of race, economic status and gender. Being mindful of how socio-geographic factors hinder the ability of marginalized persons to access quality medical care ought to be taken into account when implementing public health policies geared towards the end of cancer.

As we reach a cure for cancer, we ought to still mitigate the factors which inflate the probability of non-communicable diseases from overtaking specific segments of the population. This means ensuring that all people have access to clean air, clean water, and healthy food, ensuring that all people have access to reliable medical care and treatment. In addition, doctors ought to listen to women. Medical scientists need to study all segments of the population without defaulting to the male universal. Only when these barriers have been crossed will a scientific cure for cancer have the ability to cure all people, not just the privileged.

THE DISCOVERY OF CANCER IMMUNOTHERAPY

The immune system can be described as "an organization of cells and molecules with specialized roles in defending against infection" (Delves & Roitt, 2000). It consists of various cells with specialized functions, including phagocytes such as monocytes and macrophages, and lymphocytes such as T cells and B cells (Delves & Roitt, 2000). The body uses the immune system to interact with cells through surface receptors and classify them as either "self" or "non-self" cells (Abbott & Ustoyev, 2019). For those cells that are "non-self," the immune system will activate a response system consisting of a series of steps that can appropriately deal with the cell (Abbott & Ustoyev, 2019). Any cells that can elicit an immune response are referred to as "immunogens" (Delves & Roitt, 2000). Making use of the parts of the immune system to fight off infection is referred to as "immunotherapy" (Abbott & Ustoyev, 2019). The immune system's role in cancer has been known as early as 3000 years ago in ancient Egypt (Dobosz & Dzieciątkowski, 2019). At the time, the ancient Egyptians observed that tumours would spontaneously disappear when an individual subsequently got another infection - marked by high fever (Dobosz & Dzieciątkowski, 2019). Thus, it was clear that the immune system had the potential to control tumours. However, it wasn't until the 19th century that this promising idea would be put to the test when the immune system itself was better understood. Thus, the concept of cancer immunotherapy would first be established.

In the mid-19th century, two German scientists Wilhelm Busch and Friedrich Fehleisen observed the shrinking of tumour size after patients had been accidentally infected by erysipelas streptococcal skin infection (Dobosz & Dzieciątkowski, 2019). To further test this correlation, Busch deliberately infected a patient with erysipelas in 1868 and observed that the tumour shrank (Dobosz & Dzieciątkowski, 2019). Likewise,

Fehleisen repeated this experiment in 1882 and eventually was able to identify the bacteria directly responsible for the tumour shrinkage as *Streptococcus pyogenes* (Fehleisen, 1882).

The finding of these two German scientists was confirmed not long after by American scientist William Bradley Coley, often referred to as the "Father of Immunotherapy" (Oiseth & Aziz, 2017). Like Busch and Fehleisen, Coley observed through the retrospective study of sarcoma cases in patients that those who had been infected by erysipelas experienced a reduction in tumour size (Coley, 1893). Intrigued by this, Coley began to study this phenomenon and deliberately infected a sarcoma patient with the *Streptococcus pyogenes* bacteria in 1891 to further test it out (Coley, 1893). His experiment was successful, and the patient's tumour regressed significantly (Coley, 1893). Coley then went on to study this phenomenon through a series of experiments and eventually progressed from using the live *Streptococcus pyogenes*, to using a heat-killed strain which became known as "Coley's toxins" (Coley, 1908). He reported 1000 successful regressions in tumour size of patients who had been treated with Coley's toxins by 1908 (Coley, 1908). Unfortunately, despite initial success, Coley's toxins weren't consistent and reliable. They worked sporadically, and several other scientists who attempted to reproduce his experiments failed to do so (Oiseth & Aziz, 2017). Likewise, due to the lack of knowledge regarding how exactly the immune system worked, neither other scientists nor Coley himself could explain how and why the *Streptococcus pyogenes* worked (Dobosz & Dzieciątkowski, 2019). For this reason, his work went largely ignored for several decades.

Another breakthrough in the area of immunotherapy came around the same time, by German scientist Paul Ehrlich. He formulated the side-chain theory. His theory stated that specific cells possess side-chains on their outer surface, contributing to specific-cell recognition and antibody formation (Ehrlich, 1897). He further connected this with tumours and drew the connection that specific molecules involved in recognizing tumours could play a key role in cancer therapy (Ehrlich, 1900). His theory would serve as the base of discovering tumour-associated antigens, which would become crucial to further understanding and developing cancer immunotherapies. Through his research and knowledge in immunology, Ehrlich famously formulated the hypothesis in 1909 that the immune system could suppress tumour growth - and if it weren't for the immune system, cancer would occur at an "overwhelming frequency" (Ehrilch, 1909). Little did he know that he was planting the seeds of what would later become known as "immunosurveillance." Although, at the time, his hypothesis couldn't be proven experimentally due to a lack of technological tools, scientists over the next few decades worked to verify his hypothesis and establish the framework for cancer immunotherapy.

Further experimental evidence for Ehrlich's hypothesis came almost 50 years later, at the hands of two innovative scientists, Sir Frank Mac Farlane Burnet from Australia and Lewis Thomas from America (Parish, 2003). A lot more was understood about the immune system and its molecular components and functions at this stage. In 1949, Burnet proposed the theory of acquired immunological tolerance (Burnet & Fenner, 1949). According to this theory, lymphocytes that could respond to "self" cells during the development of the immune system in the prenatal stage were eliminated (Burnet & Fenner, 1949). This was called the immunological tolerance theory (Burnet & Fenner, 1949). This theory was revolutionary because it could explain why the immune system only responded to "non-self" cells (Burnet & Fenner, 1949). Likewise, it could explain why the immune system was incapable of responding to malignant tumour cells - since they were, in fact, the body's cells (Burnet & Fenner, 1949). However, studies conducted in the 1950s were evidence against this idea. Scientists transplanted tumours in syngeneic mice - genetically identical mice (Baldwin, 1955). They found that they were able to elicit an immune response with the addition of certain carcinogens (Baldwin, 1955). These studies denied Burnet's initial perspective that the immune system was entirely incapable of recognizing cancer cells because they were "self" cells (Parish, 2003). Instead, they revealed that there had to be some mechanism of identifying tumour cells as distinct from "self" cells (Parish, 2003). Following past research, including that of Paul Ehrlich's, there had to be tumour-associated antigens that could be recognized by the body

(Parish, 2003). Burnet believed that tumour-associated antigens could provoke an immune response that could then suppress the tumour's growth (Burnet, 1957). However, how exactly the body's immune system went about finding and recognizing these malignant cells was unclear.

Around the same time, Lewis Thomas made a revolutionary connection between transplantation and cancer, which would help Burnet in his pursuit to understand the immune response. He observed that when patients received homografts, their immune system would reject the homograft because it would identify those cells as "non-self" and attack it (Thomas, 1959). Thomas predicted that the exact mechanism responsible for rejecting the homograft must regulate neoplastic disease by eliminating new malignant cells that could form tumours (Thomas, 1959). This was a novel perspective on the relationship between cancer and the immune system. Soon after, Burnet was able to develop a more specific hypothesis. He suggested that lymphocytes constantly patrol cells and eliminate malignant cells by recognizing tumour-associated antigens (Burnet, 1967). He called this phenomenon "immunosurveillance" (Burnet, 1967). The theory of immunosurveillance, which Paul Ehrlich had first introduced, was official. For the next few years, the theory gained a lot of excitement. Much research started being conducted to understand this theory better and discover more about which tumour-associated antigens were involved in this process.

One new breakthrough in the area of transplantation that would contribute to the theory of immunosurveillance was the discovery of the immunosuppressive drug cyclosporine A (Calne et al., 1978). The purpose of this drug was to suppress the immune system to prevent it from "fighting" against the homograft (Calne et al., 1978). The drug was successful in doing just that (Calne et al., 1978). Thomas observed this and began what he called the "human experiment" to test the immunosurveillance hypothesis (Thomas, 1982). He took note of whether cancer occurred over the lifetime of thousands of transplant patients who were being treated with immunosuppressive drugs (Thomas, 1982). According to the theory, there was a much higher occurrence in those who were immunosuppressed because of the reduction in immunosurveillance in the body (Thomas, 1982). This confirmed his initial beliefs.

Although the theory of immunosurveillance started off strong, that didn't last long. Research conducted in the 1970s by Osias Stutman, an Argentinian physician, completely discredited the theory. He was working with nude mice, which lack an immune system and sought to determine the impact of having an immune system on cancer occurrence (Stutman, 1974). According to the immunosurveillance theory, nude mice should have been much more likely to develop cancer than regular mice because they would lack the mechanism of immunosurveillance (Stutman, 1974). In contrast, he found that nude mice were just as likely as standard mice to develop cancer - this meant that the immune system had no role in preventing cancer (Stutman, 1974). This research had a significant blow on the field of immunosurveillance and cancer immunotherapy. It wasn't until the late 1980s that it was discovered that nude mice did, in fact, have several lymphocytes that could escape thymic deletion - specifically T cells (Maleckar & Sherman, 1987). These could continue the process of immunosurveillance in their bodies, so nude mice weren't entirely immunodeficient (Maleckar & Sherman, 1987). This could explain the results that Stutman had observed only a decade earlier. However, the impact of Stutman's research, coupled with the difficulty the science community was having in accepting that the immune system had truly evolved to suppress tumour growth, led to negative perceptions on the theory of immunosurveillance that would last for decades to come (Parish, 2003). It wouldn't be until the turn of the century that the theory of immunosurveillance, first laid by Ehrlich and established by Burnet and Thomas, would be revived.

Another breakthrough in the area of immunotherapy was the discovery of interferon. Alick Isaacs and Jean Lindenmann released their study in 1957, which sent waves in the Science community. The study identified a molecule that could signal to the body when a virus had impacted a host cell - they called this interferon due to its interference in the function of the virus (Isaacs & Lindenmann 1957). Interferon was a cytokine molecule - a small signalling protein (Isaacs & Lindenmann 1957). This discovery was a cornerstone in understanding the body's innate immunity. It was initially only viewed as applicable against fighting viruses. However, scientists were unaware of what implications this discovery indeed had, especially in the field of cancer. In 1969, a study conducted by Ian Gresser and Chantal Bourbali drew the connection between these interferons and tumours (Gresser & Bourali 1969). Specifically, they looked at the anti-tumour effects of Interferon Type I (IFN-I), which consists of both the IFN-α and IFN-β subgroups (Gresser & Bourali 1969). They studied mice models that had been inoculated with malignant tumour cells (Gresser & Bourali 1969). The researchers found that the mice that had also been inoculated with exogenous interferon had higher survival rates than the mice that hadn't (Gresser & Bourali 1969). This revealed that IFN-I also had anti-tumour properties (Gresser & Bourali 1969). This was the first time a molecular component of the immune response to tumours had been identified. IFNs held lots of promise in the area of cancer immunotherapy. With further research in this area, scientists were eventually able to use the anti-tumour cytokine IFN-α2 as an anti-tumour treatment agent (Eno, 2017). IFN-α2 could regulate cytokines and stimulate both an innate immune response and an adaptive response (Brassard et al. 2002). This mechanism proved to be successful in many studies. In 1986, the United States Food and Drug Administration (FDA) approved IFN-α2 to be used as a cancer immuno-therapy drug (Eno, 2017). It was initially approved for hairy cell leukemia and was later expanded to be used for melanoma in 1995 (Eno, 2017). This was the first anti-tumour cytokine treatment and subsequently the first cancer immunotherapy treatment approved by the FDA.

Following the discovery of interferon, another key discovery in the area of immunology that helped progress cancer immunotherapy research was the discovery of interleukines. In 1976, Robert Gallo and his team at the United States National Institute of Health identified interleukin-2 (IL-2) as another cytokine signalling molecule that could stimulate T-cell production (Morgan et al.,1976). They did this by growing T cells in vitro and looking for potential growth factors (Morgan et al.,1976). The discovery of IL-2 was crucial to cancer immunotherapy research because it provided a direct way to ramp up the immune system in cancer (Morgan et al.,1976). In 1998, the FDA approved IL-2 as the second anti-tumour cytokine treatment, which could be used in metastatic melanoma and renal cell carcinoma (Eno, 2017).

The connection first observed by Fehleisen, Busch and Coley regarding the suppression of cancer through subsequent bacterial infections made a comeback in 1929. At the time, researchers at John Hopkins Hospital found that cancer incidence was significantly less in Tuberculosis patients than in those without TB (Pearl, 1929). A team of researchers consisting of Lloyd Old, Donald Clarke and Baruj Benacerraf found a revolutionary discovery based on this observation 30 years later. They found that the vaccine for Tuberculosis, the Bacillus Calmette-Guerin vaccine, also known as BCG, had anti-tumour properties in mice with bladder cancer (Old et al., 1959). This led to several trials being done internationally to test BCG as a potential treatment mechanism for leukemia, melanoma, lung, prostate, bladder, colon, and kidney cancer (Alcorn et al., 2015). However, the research was unsuccessful in proving BCG to be a successful treatment option for many years (Alcorn et al., 2015). Finally, in 1976, a Canadian named Alvaro Morales published a study that could successfully prove the effectiveness of BCG for use as a treatment option for bladder cancer (Morales et al., 1976). Following further trials and assessments by the National Cancer Institute, BDG became a viable treatment option. In 1990 the FDA officially approved BCG as a treatment option (Alcorn et al., 2015). BCG remains as the most commonly used immunotherapy treatment for bladder cancer globally almost 30 years later (Alcorn et al., 2015).

Lloyd Old's contributions to cancer immunotherapy didn't end there. In fact, he was a strong believer in the theory Thomas and Burnet had introduced several decades earlier. In 1977, he stated, "there is something unique about a cancer cell that distinguishes it from normal cells, and that this difference can be recognized by the body's immune system" (Old, 1977). He went on to carry out a number of studies in this field. In 2001, a team of researchers including Old, Robert Schreiber, Vijay Shankaran and Hiroaki Ikeda published a study that effectively proved that the immune system could suppress tumour formation (Shankaran et al., 2001). In particular, by looking at mice models, they found that IFN-γ and other lymphocytes were involved in the control of malignant cells (Shankaran et al., 2001). This study was revolutionary and is sometimes regarded as the revival of the cancer immunosurveillance theory. Their study also provided evidence into the mechanisms of immune recognition and demonstrated that the emergence of tumours could be through escaping immune recognition (Shankaran et al. 2001). With further studies, the concept of immunoediting was established by Old, Schrieber and Gavin Dunn in 2004. Immunoediting consisted of three phases, which were elimination, equilibrium and escape (Gavin et al., 2004). Elimination was essentially the original concept of immunosurveillance involving immune cells actively patrolling and destroying malignant cells (Gavin et al., 2004). In the equilibrium phase, there was a latent balance between the immune and malignant cells - malignant cells would neither be destroyed nor grow any larger (Gavin et al., 2004). Finally, in the escape phase, malignant cells that weren't eliminated could grow into tumours (Gavin et al., 2004). This was a dynamic process that could explain both how the immune system could suppress tumours and how tumours were able to escape destruction in their early stages (Gavin et al., 2004). Finally, following almost a century of uncertainty, the mechanism of the immune system's control of tumour growth was finally understood.

At this point, both regulating cytokine signalling molecules and BCG had proven to be successful cancer immunotherapies. Scientists began looking for even more mechanisms that could be used in cancer immunotherapies. One area of promise was checkpoint inhibitors - proteins that can block immune checkpoints. In 1995, James Allison from the University of California proposed that inhibiting CTLA-4 which is a checkpoint protein that had been discovered less than a decade prior, could potentially be used to regulate T cell activity and subsequently reduce tumour growth (Allison & Krummel 1995). Around the same time, across the globe in Japan's Kyoto University, Tasuku Honjo discovered the immune checkpoint PD-1 in 1999 (Nishimura, 1999). Over the following years, lots of research was done in the area of both these checkpoint inhibitors and very soon treatment drugs targeting each of them had been developed. In 2011, ipilimumab which was a monoclonal antibody targeting CTLA-4 became the first checkpoint inhibitor approved by the FDA for melanoma, colorectal cancer and a few others (Dobosz & Dzieciątkowski, 2019). In 2015, pembrolizumab, which was a checkpoint inhibitor for PD-1 was approved by the FDA (Dobosz v & Dzieciątkowski, 2019). It is now one of the most commonly used drugs and has since been approved for 17 different kinds of cancers (Dobosz & Dzieciątkowski, 2019).

With the further development of medical research and the onset of genetically engineering technologies, the 21st century brought a number of new and innovative cancer immunotherapies. One of these was the development of the chimeric antigen receptor T cells (CAR-T). These were developed by Michel Sadelain, Renier Brentjens, and Isabelle Rivière and their team of researchers at the Memorial Sloane Kettering Cancer Center (Maher et al., 2002). They genetically engineered CAR-T cells to target T lymphocytes to the surface of tumour cells (Maher et al., 2002). This was a very effective mechanism, and in 2017, the first CAR-T was approved by the FDA for leukemia (Dobosz v & Dzieciątkowski, 2019). Another notable discovery was the onset of oncolytic virus therapy. This entailed using viruses to treat cancer - and was a previously abandoned technique. In the 1990s, a number of researchers began looking for ways to genetically engineer viruses to make them better suited for inducing an immune response against tumours (Martuza et al., 1991). The Herpes Simplex virus type (HSV-1) was an early candidate and was engineered to induce immune responses at tumour sites (Martuza et al., 1991). In 2015, this treatment was approved for melanoma and remains the only oncolytic virus therapy approved to this day - although this technology is very promising and many other potential candidates are undergoing clinical trials (Dobosz v & Dzieciątkowski, 2019).

As technology and research progress faster than ever in the 21st century, there is optimism that the coming decades will see much progress in cancer immunotherapy treatments. Nonetheless, one cannot appreciate the scientific advances in cancer immunotherapy without acknowledging the contributions of countless researchers over the past 150 years. A revolutionary way of treating cancer that was first introduced by none other than the founding father of immunology, William Bradley Coley, has saved thousands of lives only a century later. Likewise, the contributions of many others, whether in our understanding of the immune system itself or the mechanisms involved in immunosurveillance, were crucial to the process. And these contributions have not gone unnoticed. In 2018, James Allison and Tasuku Honjo won the Nobel prize for the discovery of cancer therapy by negative immune regulation (Cancer Immunotherapy Timeline of Progress, 2021). Likewise, both were recipients of the Cancer Research Institute's highest scientific honour - the William B. Coley Award (Cancer Immunotherapy Timeline of Progress, 2021).

FATHER OF CANCER IMMUNOTHERAPY: WILLIAM BRADLEY COLEY

Also known as the "Father of Immunotherapy," William Bradley Coley was an American surgeon who made incredible contributions to cancer therapy (McCarthy, 2006). Through his investigations on the impact of bacterial infections on host immune systems and the resultant regression of tumours, he laid the foundations of immunotherapy and revolutionized cancer therapy worldwide (McCarthy, 2006).

Coley was born on January 12, 1862, in Saugatuck, Connecticut (Vernon, 2018). He was keen on his studies and very hard working from a young age, working at nearby farms for a mere $3.50/day after school (Vernon, 2018). In 1880 he started his undergraduate education at Yale University (Vernon, 2018). Upon graduation, Coley moved to Portland, Oregon, to teach Greek and Latin at Bishop Scott Government School (Vernon, 2018). After two years, he moved back and began his medical journey at Harvard Medical School (Vernon, 2018). He completed the 3-year program in just two years and graduated with his medical degree in 1888 (Vernon, 2018). Following this, he pursued an internship at New York Hospital under two of the most notable surgeons, Dr. William T Bull and Dr. Robert F Weir (Vernon, 2018). In 1890, he was presented with 17-year old Elizabeth Dashiell, who had what seemed to be a minor arm injury (Vernon, 2018). A small lump had developed on the injury site, which caused her severe pain (Vernon, 2018). No physician was able to diagnose the problem (Vernon, 2018). Coley performed a biopsy and found that she had developed a malignant tumour in her arm and was suffering from sarcoma (Vernon, 2018). He amputated her forearm to prevent further spread of the cancerous cells since this was the only available treatment at the time (Vernon, 2018). However, shortly after the amputation, Coley found that the cancerous cells had already spread to her lungs and liver (Vernon, 2018). Dashiell died on January 23, 1891, leaving a long-lasting impact on Coley (Vernon, 2018).

Thus began Coley's search for more effective cancer treatment methods. He reviewed 90 cases of sarcoma from the past 15 years at the New York Hospital and came across the miraculous case of Fred Stein from 1883 (Hall, 1997). Stein was a cancer patient with four malignant tumours on his neck (Hall, 1997). He underwent multiple surgeries, but the tumours reappeared (Hall, 1997). Shortly after the final surgery, he developed erysipelas, a common bacterial infection at the time caused by *Streptococcus pyogenes* (Hall, 1997). Within weeks, the tumour disappeared on its own, and Stein was discharged (Hall, 1997). Coley was so fascinated by this story that we went out to search for Stein and confirm that his cancer did disappear (Hall, 1997). He went door to door searching for Stein in Lower Manhattan, and after a few weeks, he was successful (McCarthy, 2006). Stein was perfectly healthy and had no evidence of cancer (McCarthy, 2006). Through this incident, Coley hypothesized that by intentionally injecting bacteria into cancer patients, he would induce tumour regression (Hall, 1997). He continued to search through literature and found 47 reported cases of bacterial infections having a beneficial impact on tumours (McCarthy, 2006). One of the first reports was from the German physician, Wilhelm Busch (McCarthy, 2006). In 1867, he reported that when a patient had contracted an erysipelas infection, their tumour suddenly disappeared (McCarthy, 2006). Following this, in 1888, another German physician known as Bruns injected a cancer patient with *Streptococcus pyogenes*, inducing erysipelas for the first time ever (McCarthy, 2006). He also reported some shrinkage of the tumour (McCarthy, 2006). With this supporting evidence, Coley was ready to test his hypothesis.

In May 1891, Coley was presented with a new patient, Signor Zola (Kienle, 2012), a 35-year old Italian man. Zola had a sarcoma of the neck and a large tumour on his tonsil, which almost completely blocked the pharynx (Kienle, 2012). This prevented him from speaking and eating and often obstructed his airway (Vernon, 2018). To test his hypothesis, Coley made small incisions on Zola and rubbed *Streptococcus pyogenes* into them every 3-4 days (Vernon, 2018). For a couple of months, he saw only slight local responses with minor shrinkage in the tumour, but it would grow back immediately (Vernon, 2018). He then decided to inject a more virulent strain of the bacteria directly into Zola's tumour to instigate a full infection (Vernon, 2018). In the first hour, Zola developed a high fever, nausea and was in pain (Kienle, 2012). Within 12 hours, the infection was in full effect (Kienle, 2012). Within 24 hours, the tumour became pale and began to dissolve (Kienle, 2012). It released a gaseous fluid for the next few days as it shrunk, and by 2 weeks it had completely disappeared (Kienle, 2012). This result was miraculous and a massive milestone from Coley.

Coley used this treatment on two more patients that year, and although there was proof of tumour shrinkage, both eventually died from the bacterial infection (McCarthy, 2006). At this point, Coley noticed a significant problem with injecting the live *Streptococcus pyogenes*: it had very inconsistent and unpredictable results (Hoption, 2003). In some cases, it was fatal; in others, the infection was too strong, causing cancer to progress even more, and yet in others, it was too difficult to induce an infection at all (Hoption, 2003). This led Coley to start searching for a safer bacteria to inject patients with, so it could instigate tumour cell death without taking too much of a toll on their overall health (McCarthy, 2006). He developed a mixture of heat-killed *Streptococcus pyogenes* and *Serratia marcescens* (McCarthy, 2006). At the time, research had shown that *Serratia marcescens* could increase the virulence of the heat-killed. So by mixing the two, he could trigger a weaker infection more consistently while not worrying about the infection being fatal (Hoption, 2003). This mixture went on to be known as Coley's Toxins (McCarthy, 2006). Coley had tried this mixture on ten patients within the next two years, with the most successful cases (McCarthy, 2006). His treatment method followed a few simple rules (Hoption, 2003). First, induce a naturally occurring infection by injecting the patient with the mixture (Hoption, 2003). The infection must come with a fever, which seemed crucial for recovery (Hoption, 2003). If the primary tumour was accessible, the injections should be made directly (Hoption, 2003). If it wasn't accessible, injections could be made intravenously or intramuscularly as well (McCarthy, 2006). For the first couple of months, injections were to be daily or every other day (Hoption, 2003). The dosage was gradually increased over time to avoid immune tolerance to it (Hoption, 2003). Once the tumour had disappeared, injections were administered weekly, for a minimum of six months (Hoption, 2003).

This was intended to help prevent the reappearance of cancer and kill any remaining cancerous cells (Hoption, 2003).

Coley received a mix of reactions from the medical community. Many traditional physicians could not understand how instigating a high fever could benefit a patient (Vernon, 2018). Others pointed out that Coley held an erroneous understanding of cancer even after it had been widely dismissed in the medical community - that tumours were caused by microorganisms (McCarthy, 2006). Thus, many physicians were repulsive of his ideas right off the bat (McCarthy, 2006). Coley faced one of the biggest obstacles was not explaining how or why his toxins worked (McCarthy, 2006). When little was known about the immune response, he could not defend his work through biological mechanisms but instead solely based on experiential evidence (McCarthy, 2006).

Nonetheless, he did receive some support from the medical community. Upon the initial release of his findings, most physicians in the USA and Europe were impressed by his discovery and celebrated his work (Vernon, 2018). Coley continued to use his toxins on patients successfully, more and more interest was ignited within the medical community (McCarthy, 2006). In 1899, the Parke Davis & Company started preparing Coley's Toxins for commercial use by physicians (McCarthy, 2006). However, as physicians began using these on patients, they found many inconsistencies in the procedures and outcomes (McCarthy, 2006). There were 13 variations of Coley's toxins, with some being more effective than others (McCarthy, 2006). In addition, Coley's records showed some cases where the mixture was injected intravenously, some intramuscularly, and some directly into the tumour (McCarthy, 2006). The effectiveness of each of these formulas and administration methods regarding particular circumstances was not tested and documented (McCarthy, 2006). Thus, many physicians did not get the same results as Coley, noticing no effect (McCarthy, 2006). In addition, Coley's toxins only seemed to be effective against sarcomas which represent only a tiny fraction of all cancers (Vernon, 2018). The inconsistencies and lack of generalizability resulted in a loss of interest not long after its commercialization (Vernon, 2018).

Moreover, around the same time was the discovery of radiation therapy for cancer (McCarthy, 2006). Due to its broad applicability, many physicians were drawn towards this treatment method instead of Coley's toxins (McCarthy, 2006). One particular physician, James Ewing, was a leading opponent to Coley's work because he firmly believed that radiation therapy was the best option for treating sarcomas (McCarthy, 2006). Ewing was the most famous cancer pathologist in the US and senior to Coley at the Memorial Hospital (McCarthy, 2006). Ewing prohibited Coley from using his toxins at the hospital, despite their success in the majority of Coley's previous work (McCarthy, 2006).

In 1920, a leading surgeon named Ernest Amory Codman set on a mission to create the first Bone Sarcoma Registry - a collection of diagnoses and treatments for bone cancers across the country to standardize it (McCarthy, 2006). He invited Ewing and other prominent physicians to assist with this project (McCarthy, 2006). Together they evaluated bone cancer cases from across the country (McCarthy, 2006). Unfortunately, many of Coley's cases were not accepted into the registry because they did not assume that the toxins were effective (McCarthy, 2006). Codman argued that the successful results reported by Coley were not a result of the toxins but instead due to incorrect diagnoses (McCarthy, 2006). Despite the backlash, Coley remained firm in his stance and continued to use his toxins on patients (McCarthy, 2006). Finally, in a symposium in 1935, Codman took back his words and admitted that Coley's toxins did have some degree of effectiveness (McCarthy, 2006).

Coley's career came to an end upon his death on April 16, 1936. However, he managed to treat nearly 1000 patients with his toxins throughout his lifetime and published over 150 papers (McCarthy, 2006). His two children, Bradley and Helen, carried his legacy until the 21st century (McCarthy, 2006). Bradley became the head of the Bone Tumour Service at the Memorial Hospital, succeeding his father (McCarthy, 2006). In 1948, he published a textbook on bone tumours in which he supported the use of Coley's toxins as a part of therapy (McCarthy, 2006). Helen became a cancer researcher (McCarthy, 2006). She analyzed her father's work and studied his toxins in more depth (McCarthy, 2006). She found that nearly half of his cases had close to full tumour regression, and many of his reports were significantly better than the popular treatments used at the time (McCarthy, 2006). Coley's toxins were clinically proven on a large scale, but Helen had a hard time bringing this reality to the medical community's attention (Vernon, 2018).

By this time, radiotherapy had been well established (Hoption, 2003). Chemotherapy had just been discovered and was gaining widespread acceptance and popularity fast (Hoption, 2003). Both of these treatments were more accessible, easy to comprehend, and could be standardized (Hoption, 2003). They both used a similar immunosuppressive approach, which countered the entire concept of immunotherapy (Hoption, 2003). Thus, many lost interest in Coley's toxins and preferred one of these treatment approaches (Hoption, 2003). In 1952, the Parke Davis & Company stopped selling Coley's toxins for commercial use (McCarthy, 2006). In 1963, the US Food and Drug Administration assigned Coley's toxins a "new drug" status, refusing to acknowledge it as a proven drug despite its use for nearly 70 years (Hoption, 2003). With this status, one would need to go through an extremely expensive procedure to test and prove that the drug worked, before being granted permission to use it (Hoption, 2003). As a result, it became nearly impossible to use the drug for cancer treatment in the country (McCarthy, 2006). In addition, in 1965, the American Cancer Society put Coley's toxins on the "Unproven Methods of Cancer Management" blacklist, neglecting his research once again (McCarthy, 2006).

In 1953, Helen started the Cancer Research Institute (CRI), through which she continued her research on Coley's toxins (Vernon, 2018). The mission statement of this institute was "...understanding the immune system and its relationship to cancer" (Vernon, 2018). Another physician named Lloyd J Old, from the Sloan Kettering Cancer Research Institute, eventually joined the CRI as the medical and scientific director (Vernon, 2018). His research pertained to microbes and endotoxins, and he had an interest in immunotherapy (Vernon, 2018). Together Helen and Old were able to convince the American Cancer Society to remove Coley's toxins from their "Unproven Methods of Cancer Management" blacklist, allowing for further development of immunotherapy using Coley's toxins (Vernon, 2018). Thus, research in cancer immunotherapy continued for the next few decades.

In 1998 a physician named Bruce Beutler and his colleagues made a ground-breaking discovery in understanding immunotherapy at the Scripps Institute in La Jolla, CA, USA (Vernon, 2018). They found that bacterial toxin lipopolysaccharides can activate toll-like receptors, a specific type of immune system cells (Vernon, 2018). Toll-like receptors can then initiate a response from the immune system and kill the tumour cells (Vernon, 2018). This finding demonstrated that when Coley injected the patients with bacteria, the bacteria were able to initiate an immune system response and dissolve the tumours (Vernon, 2018). The fever that occurred was a mechanism used by the immune system to initiate an effective immune response (Vernon, 2018). Thus, Coley's theory was confirmed (Vernon, 2018).

As we entered the 21st century, immunotherapy research and our fundamental understanding of the immune system progressed. Coley's work finally received its recognition and became the cornerstone for advancements in the field. The CRI has been a leading institute in cancer research, funding and conducting some groundbreaking research in the area (Vernon, 2018). In 1975, the CRI established the William B. Coley Award for Distinguished Research in Basic and tumour Immunology, to be awarded to researchers who have furthered our understanding of the immune system and the development of cancer immunotherapy (*William B. Coley Award*, 2020). Receipts are awarded a medal and a cash prize of $5,000 (*William B. Coley Award*, 2020). To date, over 85 people have received his award (*William B. Coley Award*, 2020). Although Coley faced much criticism in his lifetime, he left an incredible legacy that has revolutionized our understanding of biology and been a means through which hundreds of thousands of lives were and continue to be saved. He was indeed a man before his time and will long be recognized in the scientific community.

CANCER AND THE HOST IMMUNE SYSTEM

Cancer is a disease that has been present in our society for a long time. Unfortunately, it has been steadily increasing in prevalence, and thus, people's awareness of cancer has also increased. We have reached a point where it is safe to say that everyone will know someone who has been impacted by cancer. On top of that, cancer is one of the leading causes of death in many places worldwide, including Canada. Copious amounts of research have gone into finding treatments and cures for cancer and understanding how and why cancer might originate and invade the body. To understand this, we have to look at the immune system responsible for protecting the body from parasites, pathogens, and other illnesses. One thing that is crucial to understand is how cancer evades the immune system and how the immune system reacts to cancerous cells. Once this is understood, research can begin to look at how the immune system could be activated to rid the body of cancer and how the immune system reacts to various cancer treatments.

First, to understand how cancer interacts with the immune system, we will briefly go over the different components of the immune system and how they function. The human immune system has three main features: each plays an essential role in protecting and keeping the body healthy (Zavitz, 2021). These components are the intrinsic barriers, innate immunity, and adaptive immune response (Zavitz, 2021).

The first line of defence is the intrinsic barriers present to prevent infection from entering the body. There are four types of intrinsic barriers: mechanical, chemical, microbiological and physiological (Zavitz, 2021). The mechanical barriers can be things such as expulsive forces to eliminate pathogens, such as coughing, sneezing, defecation or urination, ciliary beating, which will move mucus to the mouth to allow pathogens to be swallowed, and tighten junctions in the epithelium, so pathogens cannot sneak in (Zavitz, 2021). These immune system components usually do not play a huge role in cancer, but they are still essential to know. There are also chemical barriers, such as having a low pH in the stomach to denature pathogens or having proteolytic enzymes, such as lysozyme and pepsin, to denature proteins (Zavitz, 2021). Microbiological barriers can be commensal flora to compete with pathogens for nutrients that they both need (Zavitz, 2021). Finally, the last type of intrinsic barrier is physiological barriers such as temperature regulation. This can be helpful for the immune response as pathogens that often live at room temperature cannot live at body temperature (Zavitz, 2021).

Next, we will discuss another part of the human immune system: innate immunity. The natural immune response consists of preformed cells, meaning that it has an immediate reaction (Zavitz, 2021). Some other vital things to note about the innate immune system are that it is activated when Pattern Recognition Receptors (PRR) on our cells recognize Pathogen Associated Molecular Patterns (PAMP) invaders (Zavitz, 2021). Since the PRR are encoded in our germline, they are not variable and have broad cross-reactivity across pathogens (Zavitz, 2021). Finally, innate immunity contains no memory component, but it will also never bind to the body's proteins (Zavitz, 2021). Some essential innate immune cells in the body are macrophages, neutrophils, dendritic cells, natural killer cells, mast cells, eosinophils and basophils (Zavitz, 2021). Macrophages are cells that can phagocytose, or in other words, ingest bacteria and dead cells (Zavitz, 2021). They can also produce cytokines, which are small molecules that establish the inflammatory response (Zavitz, 2021). Macrophages are sentinel cells, which means that they are present in healthy tissue and are recruited to sites of infection as needed (Zavitz, 2021). Moving on to neutrophils, these are granulated cells, which means that they contain toxic granules that can kill invaders (Zavitz, 2021). They are recruited to sites where inflamed tissues are present through chemokines, a subset of cytokines (Zavitz, 2021). One important thing to note is that the toxic granules that neutrophils contain are not only harmful to invaders but are also toxic to humans and therefore have to be closely regulated to prevent the adverse effects of immunopathology (Zavitz, 2021). Dendritic cells are also phagocytes. However, these cells play a role in activating the adaptive immune response, which will be touched upon later. It is essential to understand that these cells are antigen-presenting cells which means that they pick up tiny pathogens and bring them to the lymph nodes to activate T-cells and B-cells (Zavitz, 2021). Moving on to natural killer cells, which are cells that kill virus-infected cells and mutated cells (Zavitz, 2021). They do this by releasing cytotoxic granules that cause cells to rupture or undergo apoptosis (Zavitz, 2021). These cells can play an essential role in preventing cancer, as they work to kill cells that have undergone mutations before they can reproduce and spread throughout the body (Zavitz, 2021). Mast cells are cells found in the mucosa and are important in allergic reactions due to them releasing histamine. This can cause various responses to protect the body, such as causing diarrhea to expel the pathogen (Zavitz, 2021). These cells, along with eosinophils, can help battle parasites and play a role in protecting mucosal surfaces (Zavitz, 2021). It is therefore unsurprising that both mast cells and eosinophils are found along the GI tract (Zavitz, 2021). Finally, we have basophils which are also crucial in allergic reactions (Zavitz, 2021). Basophils also play a role in blood clotting by releasing heparin (Zavitz, 2021).

Innate immunity will initially battle pathogens and mutated cells in our bodies responsible for getting the threat under control. However, without the adaptive immune response kicking in 3-5 days later, many threats would not be completely cleared (Zavitz, 2021). Activating the adaptive immune response is where the dendritic cells that were mentioned earlier come into play. When the dendritic cells go to the lymph nodes with viral antigens (which are molecules to which antibodies can specifically bind) on their surface, T-cells become activated. T-cells are a vital part of the immune system (Zavitz, 2021). There are several different types of T-cells:

There are the CD8+ cytotoxic T-cells responsible for killing infected cells and preventing the pathogen or infection from spreading and reproducing (Zavitz, 2021).

There are also CD4+ helper T-cells responsible for causing cytotoxic T-cells to proliferate and differentiate, as well as being responsible for activating B-cells, another component of the adaptive immune system (Zavitz, 2021).

B-cells are cells responsible for secreting antibodies, which can help the body fight against pathogens. Antibodies can help in several different ways (Zavitz, 2021). They can perform neutralization, where the antibodies will coat the pathogen and prevent it from binding to the epithelium (Zavitz, 2021). They can also partake in opsonization, which can be thought of as the antibodies tagging the pathogen so that phagocytes can recognize it and eliminate it through phagocytosis (Zavitz, 2021). B-cells can also differentiate into resting memory cells, which have a lifespan as long as a human lifespan (Zavitz, 2021). These cells provide humans with immunity to a pathogen or virus after clearing it for the first time (Zavitz, 2021).

While the human immune system is infinitely more complicated than mentioned above, understanding the basic principles of the immune system is essential to understanding what goes wrong in the immune system that allows cancer to occur. Before moving on to how cancer evades the immune system, here is a brief overview of cancer. There are many different types of cancer, but they all occur when the body's cells begin to divide without stopping (National Cancer Institute [NCI], 2007). In a healthy body, cells will grow and divide to form new cells as they need them, while old and damaged cells will die. However, cancer cells are a problem because they ignore the signals that usually tell cells to stop dividing or the signals that begin apoptosis, otherwise known as programmed cell death (NCI, 2007). Apoptosis is the usual mechanism the body uses to get rid of unneeded cells. Not only are cancer cells able to continue to multiply and evade these signals, but they also can induce nearby normal cells to create a hospitable microenvironment (NCI, 2007). This includes causing normal cells to form blood vessels that will supply the cancerous cells with oxygen and nutrients and remove waste products (NCI, 2007). This allows the cancerous cells to continue to multiply and form tumours. As these cells continue to multiply, they will begin to invade nearby tissues and interfere with how those tissues function (NCI,

2007). Furthermore, cancer cells can break away from where they first were formed and travel through the blood or the lymph system to form new tumours called metastatic tumours in other parts of the body (NCI, 2007). However, why does the immune system not attack and eliminate cancer cells? We discussed earlier how the immune system could eradicate mutated cells, so how does cancer evade it?

The process of cancer evading the immune system is complex and includes many variables. The immune system is usually able to destroy cancer cells because cancer cells present tumour antigens. This alerts the immune system that these cells need to be eliminated (Vinay et al., 2015). The cytotoxic T cells and the helper T cells will curb cancer development using various mechanisms (Vinay et al., 2015). However, due to the genetic instability and the constant tumour cell division, many of the cells can evade the immune system. This leads to a type of equilibrium, where the cancer cells continue to divide (Vinay et al., 2015). Some are eliminated due to the immune system recognizing the tumour antigens on the cells, while others evade elimination. During this period, the tumour often appears dormant, as it does not grow but instead stays a regular size and is not eliminated (Vinay et al., 2015). Unfortunately, as this process continues, the immune system will eventually begin to be unable to eradicate the cancerous cells either because of immune-suppressive effects or the loss of target antigen expression (Vinay et al., 2015). When this occurs, the tumour starts to proliferate, which is called tumour escape. This is often when clinical symptoms of cancer begin to present, as the tumour is now big enough to invade surrounding tissues and negatively impact those tissues' function (Vinay et al., 2015).

There are several immune suppressive effects that cancer uses to evade the immune system. One of the essential mechanisms of tumour immune escape is suppressive cells in the tumour microenvironment. A significant type of suppressive cell in the tumour microenvironment is regulatory T cells (Vinay et al., 2015). Evidence shows that tumour-derived regulatory T cells have higher suppressive activity than naturally occurring regulatory T cells (Vinay et al., 2015). Furthermore, regulatory T cells are also drawn to the tumour microenvironment by tumour cell-mediated chemokine production (Vinay et al., 2015). Another mechanism of having regulatory T cells present around the cancerous cells is that transforming growth factor-beta (TGF-β) can convert cytotoxic T cells, which work to eliminate the tumour, into suppressive T- regulatory cells (Vinay et al., 2015). Since tumour cells produce TGF-β, they will also be present in the tumour microenvironment (Vinay et al., 2015). Considering that all these factors are present together in the tumour microenvironment, it is unsurprising that tumours are very good at immunosuppression, which allows them to survive and continue to grow.

Besides regulatory T-cells, there are a variety of other immunosuppressive mediators. These mediators include suppressive cytokines, such as IL-8, IL-10 and tumour necrosis factor-α (TNF-α) (Vinay et al., 2015). These mediators are produced either by the cancer cells or by other cells present in the tumour microenvironment. These cells also have factors that can inhibit the differentiation of dendritic cells (Vinay et al., 2015). Without dendritic cells, the immune system will be less able to efficiently present tumour antigens to the adaptive immune system in the lymph nodes (Vinay et al., 2015). Without this step, the adaptive immune system will be less able to target the cancerous tumour cells, which will therefore be able to continue to differentiate and multiply.

However, immune suppression is not the only way that tumours evade the immune system. They are also able to avoid immune surveillance by down-regulating the expression of tumour antigen. This means that the immune system will be less able to recognize the tumour, and thus, the cytotoxic T cells will not recognize the tumour as a target (Vinay et al., 2015). This mechanism focuses less on suppressing the immune system and more on the cancerous tumour cells avoiding detection from the immune system.

Finally, tumour cells also frequently do not express costimulatory molecules. Without the costimulatory molecules, tumour cells can interact with the T-cell receptor without being eliminated (Vinay et al., 2015). This is because without costimulation, engaging the T-cell receptor will not be fatal to the cancerous cell (Vinay et al., 2015).

However, even with all these mechanisms in place to suppress the immune system and avoid immunosurveillance, cells in the tumour will be able to be targeted by the human immune system, often because they have receptors that the ligands of natural killer cells can target; the tumour deals with these cells through apoptosis, otherwise known as programmed cell death (Vinay et al., 2015). This will down-regulate cells with these receptors, which means that the receptors will be present in smaller quantities on the tumour (Vinay et al., 2015). Having fewer of these receptors on the tumour prevents the tumour from further damage from the ligands of natural killer cells, allowing it to avoid the attack of the innate immune cells (Vinay et al., 2015).

All these mechanisms work together to help cancerous cells avoid immune detection and elimination, allowing them to continue to grow and become clinically significant. However, due to the advancement of modern medicine, there are now many available treatments for cancer. Most of these treatments affect the immune system either by directly activating the immune system to eliminate the cancerous cells or through a more indirect path.

One thing that is important to be aware of is that cancer can increase infection risk by itself. It can do this in a variety of different ways, depending on the type of cancer. For example, cancers that start in the immune system blood cells, such as lymphomas, multiple myeloma, and leukemia, can alter these immune cells and interfere with their ability to protect the body ("Why People With Cancer," n.d.). Another issue can be if the cancer cells get into the bone marrow, where blood cells are made. Once the cancerous cells are in the bone marrow, they can destroy normal bone marrow cells so that not enough healthy bone marrow cells will be left to make white blood cells (leukocytes) ("Why People With Cancer", n.d.). Without these cells, the body will be at higher risk of contracting and suffering from infections and pathogens, and the immune system will not be functioning at a high enough level to fight infection. Other types of cancer, such as tumours that grow on the skin or mucous membranes, can damage the intrinsic immune barriers ("Why People With Cancer", n.d.). These tumours can break these barriers, which gives germs and pathogens a chance to enter the body. Tumours could also lead to various other problems, such as reducing blood flow to areas of the body or blocking mucus drainage, which could lead to infections ("Why People With Cancer", n.d.).

One of the most common and well-known treatments for cancer is chemotherapy. Chemotherapy will target and eliminate rapidly growing cells, such as cancer cells. However, it does not discriminate between cancer cells and rapidly-growing healthy cells, such as hair, blood and bone marrow cells ("Why People With Cancer", n.d.). However, since healthy cells can repair damage much better than cancerous cells, once the chemotherapy treatment ends, healthy cells should recover to similar levels to what they were before the therapy ("Why People With Cancer", n.d.). In contrast, the cancerous cells should be eradicated. Despite this, while chemotherapy is being administered, it will damage the bone marrow. This will make the bone marrow less able to produce red blood cells, white blood cells and platelets. Since white blood cells, otherwise known as leukocytes, are an essential part of the immune system, having fewer of them will harm the immune system. One type of white blood cell often particularly affected is the neutrophil ("Why People With Cancer", n.d.). Chemotherapy will decrease the number of neutrophils in your blood, which can cause neutropenia ("Why People With Cancer", n.d.). This will result in the body not fighting infections the same way it could before the chemotherapy. The severity of damage that chemotherapy causes the immune system will depend on the type of chemotherapy offered and the dose, frequency, and duration of treatment ("Why People With Cancer", n.d.). However, after the treatment is over, blood cell and immune blood cell counts should return to normal levels after some time has passed.

Another standard treatment option for those with cancer is radiation therapy. Radiation therapy will use high-energy waves, such as X-rays and gamma rays, to destroy or damage cancer cells ("How Radiation Therapy", n.d.). The radiation will damage the DNA inside the cancer cells, which will prevent them from growing and dividing and can even cause the cancer cells to die ("How Radiation Therapy", n.d.). Radiation is a more local treatment than chemotherapy, so only the cancerous cells and nearby healthy cells should be affected. One of the goals of radiation is to try to damage the cancer cells while causing minimal harm to nearby healthy cells ("How Radiation Therapy", n.d.). However, radiation can still cause low white blood cell counts, especially if total body irradiation (TBI) is administered ("How Radiation Therapy", n.d.). Total body irradiation is where the whole body is treated with radiation, so it can be especially likely to cause low leukocyte counts ("How Radiation Therapy", n.d.).

An alternative procedure that is often used in patients with cancer is surgery. Surgery is often used to remove a tumour or repair damage caused by cancerous cells ("Why People With Cancer", n.d.). Any type of major surgery can pose a risk to the immune system. One reason for this is because the surgery involves opening the body up and breaking through the skin ("Why People With Cancer", n.d.). This can allow germs and pathogens a pathway to get into the body and let an infection take hold ("Why People With Cancer", n.d.). Furthermore, surgery is a very invasive procedure that weakens the immune system while the body recovers ("Why People With Cancer", n.d.). Finally, depending on what was removed during surgery, there may be lasting effects on the immune system. For example, removing lymph nodes or the spleen can cause the immune system to be weakened in the long term because these tissues and organs played an essential role in the immune system ("Why People With Cancer", n.d.).

Another type of cancer therapy that directly involves the immune system is immunotherapy. Immunotherapy aims to have the immune system recognize and attack the cancer cells ("How Immunotherapy is Used", n.d.). However, this can be challenging due to all the mechanisms cancer cells have to evade the immune system. To overcome this, immunotherapy will target the immune system to help it target cancer cells with greater accuracy and strength. An example of a cancer immunotherapy treatment is checkpoint inhibitors. These are drugs that will inhibit some of the immune system's checkpoints that are in place to prevent immune cells from attacking the body's cells ("How Immunotherapy is Used", n.d.). Removing these checkpoints can help the immune system successfully recognize and eliminate cancer cells ("How Immunotherapy is Used", n.d.). Another type of immunotherapy is cancer vaccines. Like vaccines that prevent viral infections, cancer vaccines will put substances into the body to start an immune response against cancer. ("How Immunotherapy is Used", n.d.) Monoclonal antibodies can also be given. These can be thought of as immune system proteins that are synthesized in a lab ("How Immunotherapy is Used", n.d.). This means that they can be designed to attack very specific cells, such as a particular part of a cancer cell ("How Immunotherapy is Used", n.d.). Finally, chimeric antigen receptor T-cell therapy can also be used. This involves taking some of the cancer patient's T-cells and mixing them with a virus that will allow the T-cells to learn how to attach to tumour cells ("How Immunotherapy is Used", n.d.). When these T-cells are returned to the patient's body, they will now be able to find and eliminate the cancer cells ("How Immunotherapy is Used", n.d.).

Cancer and cancer treatments can have a significant effect on the immune system. Cancer interacts with all three components of the immune system (intrinsic barriers, innate immunity and adaptive immunity) and has many complex strategies and survival mechanisms that suppress the immune system and allows it to avoid immune surveillance. Furthermore, cancer can also decrease the number of leukocytes and neutrophils in the immune system and damage the intrinsic barriers, which leaves the body more vulnerable to infection and pathogens. Many life-saving cancer treatments also can damage and weaken the immune system, though luckily, these effects are reversible. Finally, immunotherapy, one of the more recent promising new cancer treatments, can prime the immune system to attack and eliminate cancer cells. Considering all this, it is evident that understanding the immune system is necessary for developing new cancer treatments and understanding the effect cancer has on the body. After all, what better way to fight unwanted mutated cancer cells than by using the body's own defence system.

WHAT IS CANCER IMMUNOTHERAPY?

Immunotherapy was pioneered by New York surgeon William B. Coley who created a vaccination composed of a mixture of attenuated strepto-coccal and staphylococcal bacteria to treat sarcoma (Schuster et al., 2006). Coley began an injection made of a non-harmful hemolytic pathogen. The vaccination aimed to treat a malignant tumour. A short time later, immu-nologists Lewis Thomas and Mac Farlane Burnet developed the concept of cancer immunosurveillance. Since the function of the immune system is to protect from cancer and maintain tissue homeostasis (Fisher, P. B. et al., 2019). Cancer immunosurveillance aims to prevent tumour development by early targeting abnormal cells by the host's immune system (Schuster et al., 2006, Bagherifar et al., 2021). These concepts set a foundation for modern immunotherapy. Current research in the Journal of Nanobio-technology describes cancer immunotherapy as a cancer treatment that aims to improve antitumour immune responses (Bagherifar et al., 2021). Furthermore, immunotherapy is typically used in combination with the current treatment methods, such as chemotherapy, radiation and surgery.

In contrast to the traditional treatment methods, immunotherapy har-nesses the immune system to battle cancer cells and has demonstrated an increase in overall survival rate in preclinical studies. Immunotherapy is a general term for treatment methods that are classified into active and passive. Each method is conducted based on the state of the host immune system and the mechanism of immunotherapeutic agents (Bagherifar et al., 2021). In other words, the method of immunotherapeutic treatment is influenced by how well the immune system is able to incorporate treat-ment methods. One of the promising cancer immunotherapy strategies is utilizing immunomodulators. The immunomodulation is based on stimulating the function of T cells by blocking or activating regulatory receptors using antibodies, which prevents the progression of cancer. Recently, antibody-based immunotherapy has shifted to targeting immune cells instead of cancer cells. T cells are a specific type of white blood cell called lymphocytes. In cancer immunotherapy, T cells have a cardinal role in the annihilation of cancer cells. Efficacious immunomodulatory antibodies target the PD-1, PD-L1 and CTLA-4 inhibitory receptors on the surface of T cells and, by binding to them, activate antitumour T cells to destroy tumour cells. Programmed cell death protein 1 (PD-1) and programmed cell death 1 ligand 1 (PD-L1) play an essential role in regulating the immune system (Bagherifar et al., 2021). Further, the Journal of Immunology explains the aim of CTLA-4 as an inhibitory immune checkpoint receptor is to slow down the rapid reproduction of T cells by outcompeting a secondary immune cell signal (Koury et al., 2018).

The host's immune system recognizes cancer by identifying tumour-specific antigens or tumour-associated antigens. Antigens are any foreign substances that cause an immune response, and tumour-specific antigens are unique to cancer cells. In contrast to tumour-specific antigens, tumour-associated antigens are expressed in various ways depending on the specific elements of the cancer cells relative to normal cells (Koury et al., 2018). During the growth of a tumour, tumour cells display abnormal protein-like tumour-associated antigens. In addition, metastatic cells learn to invade the surrounding healthy tissue causing the disease to spread. The metastatic cells, which are secondary cancer cells, break away from the origin point of the tumour and spread throughout the host's body. (Schuster et al., 2006). To infect the host, metastatic cells grow and become tumours that are incredibly invasive and capable of dodging the immune checkpoints responsible for regulating the immune system (Kruger et al., 2019). Therefore, immune system checkpoints monitor the immune system's strength and moderate any possible tissue damage due to the immune responses. Immune system checkpoints do this by changing the immune response to damage (Koury et al., 2018). However, cancer cells can conceal themselves from the immune system checkpoints. Cancer immunotherapy aims to restore the reactivity of the host's immune system to combat cancer (Schuster et al., 2006). Hence, checkpoint inhibitors are a class of immunotherapies that induce a T-cell propitiated antitumour response by selectively blocking inhibitory checkpoint receptors that are vulnerable to manipulation by cancer cells (Koury et al., 2018).

Immune checkpoint inhibitors are tumour-specific monoclonal antibodies (mAbs) that target immune checkpoint molecules and activate anti-tumour resistance for various serious illnesses, such as prostate and pancreatic cancers, metastatic melanoma, renal cell carcinoma (RCC) and non-small cell lung cancer (Bagherifar et al., 2021). MAbs are engineered to bind to tumour-specific antigens and can be used alone or reversibly combined with specific medications, toxins, or radioactive agents and carry them to cancer cells. The first checkpoint inhibitor approved for clinical use was called ipilimumab. Ipilimumab was created to target the immune checkpoint cytotoxic T lymphocyte-associated antigen 4 (CTLA-4) and garnished a fair amount of success (Kruger et al., 2019). Anti- CTLA-4 releases the natural slowing down of T-cell production, allowing them to function for an extended period. The anti-CTLA-4 therapies increase the immune system's antitumour response by blocking the CTLA-4 receptors that allow T-cell production.

In addition to the anti-CTLA-4 treatment, anti-PD-1/PD-L1 treatment is a checkpoint inhibitor of the primary focus of cancer immunotherapies. PD-1 and PD-L1 play an essential role in regulating the immune system and checkpoint inhibitors that target them. By 2018, Anti-PD-1/PD-L1 therapies had significantly positive outcomes in more than 15 types of cancer in clinical trials (Koury et al., 2018). Stopping the invasion of cancerous cells with checkpoint inhibitors can cause long-lasting remissions in numerous cancer types, such as melanoma and lung cancer (Kruger et al., 2019). Moreover, immunotherapy is less toxic on healthy cells, reducing the unfavourable effects of traditional therapies (Bagherifar et al., 2021).

Active cancer immunotherapy aims to introduce an increasing, long-lasting tumour antigen-specific immune response. In other words, active immunotherapy seeks to produce long-term improvements in the host's immune system, allowing the immune system to recognize and attack the cancer cells (Schuster et al., 2006). To establish tumour-associated antigens, materials are obtained from a biopsy of the tumour. Then, the immune response against the tumour can be improved by stimulating the immune system using an imitation response created from the tumour biopsy. (Schuster et al., 2006). Active immunotherapy involves in vivo activation of the host's immune system by stimulating effector cell functions. In vivo immunotherapy requires the treatment explicitly to take place within the host. Therefore, active immunotherapy aims to induce cancer cell death with different anti-cancer vaccines such as peptide vaccines, whole-cell vaccines, and dendritic cell-based vaccines (Bagherifar et al., 2021).

In addition to introducing an immune response by administering a tumour antigen as a vaccine, treatment methods include dendritic cells obtained from the host. Discovered in 1973 by Dr. Ralph Steinman and his colleagues, dendritic cells are produced in the bone marrow and play an essential part in the induction and regulation of the immune system. Reapplication of the dendritic cells is used to break the host's immune tolerance for tumour-associated antigens (Schuster et al., 2006, Zhang et al., 2021). Dendritic cells play an essential role in the initial activation of cancer-reactive T-cells. Specifically, dendritic cells are found in submucosal and lymphoid tissues (such as tissues in the airway and intestine) and throughout the body. Further, they serve as sensors against foreign substances (bacteria, fungi, viruses) that enter the body (Zhang et al., 2021). Dendritic cells will invade foreign bodies to move through the lymphatic vessels and into the draining lymph nodes.

During this process, the dendritic cells are activated, and antigen-presenting and co-stimulatory molecules are upregulated to stimulate T-cells. This process is the first event in the acquired immune response (Zhang et al., 2021). Dendritic cell vaccinations are prepared with cancer antigen-loaded dendritic cells, which activate cancer-reactive T cells. This method is considered more dependable than administering cancer antigen-derived compounds alone or viral vectors expressing cancer antigens or directly helping inactivated cancer cells. (Zhang et al., 2021). The presentation of tumour-associated antigens through the host's antigen-presenting cells to the host's T-Cells is an essential requirement for increased immunity against tumour antigens, rather than direct activation of T-cells (Schuster et al., 2006). Since cancer cells do not present any evidence they are dangerous at the early stages, the immune system does not respond to tumour antigens. Therefore, the dendritic cell vaccine stimulates anti-tumour immune responses in cancer patients to correct the immune system, thereby producing efficient antigen-specific T cells (Bagherifar et al., 2021).

By 2006, a large body of data had been collected using whole tumour cells as the source of tumour antigens for vaccination. Genetic modification of tumour cells has widely been used to provide danger signals necessary for efficient activation of antigen-presenting cells, leading to T-cell stimulation (Schuster et al., 2006). Today, combining the dendritic cell vaccine with other immunotherapy agents has been used successfully in several clinical studies (Bagherifar et al., 2021). Several cancer vaccines have been studied, many of which are intended to induce a tumour-specific immune response. In general, cancer vaccines can be divided into two forms; either protein- or polypeptide-containing vaccines. In other words, vaccines are either whole-cell cancer vaccines or viral vector vaccines. In most approaches, the immunization antigens must be combined with solid adjuvants or cytokines to generate an immune response (Schuster et al., 2006). In other words, the vaccinations are mixed with a solid substance to improve the immune response or small protein cells familiar to the immune system.

Passive cancer immunotherapy provides a tumour antigen-specific immune response by supplying massive amounts of effector molecules (Schuster et al., 2006). Passive cancer immunotherapy can be antibody-based, in which case it creates a link between tumour-associated antigens and the host's immune system by providing tumour antigen-specific antibodies (Schuster et al., 2006). Furthermore, passive immunotherapy uses immunotherapeutic agents such as cytokines and tumour-specific monoclonal antibodies (mAbs). Immune activation is at the forefront of cancer immunotherapy and plays a role via several immune stimulants such as cytokines and agonists. Cytokines have several functions, including induction of dendritic cell maturation, proliferation and activation of T cells. Cytokines regulate both the cells of the innate immune system and the adaptive immune system. Cytokines cause resistant cell growth and differentiation. Further, they regulate inflammatory or anti-inflammatory responses in various cell types (Bagherifar et al., 2021). Cytokines are able to function following the binding to their respective receptors on the target cells (Schuster et al., 2006). Some cytokines can kill tumour cells by providing signals that discourage growth and encourage the death of harmful cells (Bagherifar et al., 2021).

In addition to cytokines and mAbs, the most effective modern approach to immunotherapeutic is adoptive cell transfer therapy (ACT), also known as cellular immunotherapy. The three forms of ACT that have been developed for cancer therapy include tumour-infiltrating T lymphocyte (TIL), chimeric antigen receptor (CAR) T cell, and engineered T cell receptor (Bagherifar et al., 2021). Adoptive T cell transfers and bivalent antibodies are immunotherapies that induce a T cell-mediated antitumour response by selectively blocking the inhibitory checkpoint receptors subject to manipulation by cancer cells (Koury et al., 2018). ACT involves isolating a cancer patient's tumour-specific lymphocytes, a type of small white blood cell, ex-vivo modification, activation and expansion, and subsequently, their reinfusion to the patient (Bagherifar et al., 2021). Tumour-specific Lymphocytes are extracted from the host and engineered external to the host to express artificial T cell receptors. As a result, the tumour-specific lymphocytes gain the ability to target the cancer cells (Bagherifar et al., 2021). Together, the immunotherapeutic agents enhance the body's immune response to an antigen, optimizing the host's immune system to efficiently fight tumour cells rather than inducing cancer cell death (Bagherifar et al., 2021). mAbs based cancer therapies have shown significant clinical responses in treating hematological malignancies and solid cancers. Specifically, Rituximab was the first mAb approved for use in passive cases of lymphomas (Schuster et al., 2006). Adoptive T cell transfers and bivalent antibodies are checkpoint inhibitors.

Moreover, T cells originate in the thymus gland and are essential in the immune response, and bivalent antibodies are self-cloning cells that recognize cancer cells in the host. In general, a simple contrast between active and passive cancer immunotherapy is to note that active immunotherapy creates long-lasting immunity. In contrast, passive cancer immunotherapy is short-lived and dependent on repeated applications (Schuster et al., 2006). There are a large number of clinically approved immunotherapy treatments. For example, in breast cancer cases, immunotherapy is under consideration as a new mode of therapy in combination with traditional treatment methods. In breast tumours, immune checkpoint regulators are presented in large numbers and play a significant role in immunotherapy resistance in the host (Fisher, P. B. et al., 2019). As previously mentioned, cell death protein-1 (PD-1) and cytotoxic T-lymphocyte-associated protein-4 (CTLA-4) are two major immune checkpoint molecules that have been studied extensively in terms of cancer immunotherapy. While the development of breast cancer is strongly linked to genetic and epigenetic aspects of tumour development, the role of the immune system in tumour development, progression and eventual metastasis cannot be overlooked. Carcinogen-induced breast cancer has been shown to correlate with tumour development, proliferation and severe impairment of immune response (Fisher, P. B. et al., 2019).

Immune checkpoints are a significant concern for cancer immunotherapy due to their role in limiting cytotoxic T cell activity and antitumour immune response. Together, the expression of multiple checkpoint markers in breast cancer suggests the combination of more than one checkpoint inhibitor or the combination with other immunotherapeutic strategies could offer an increased therapeutic effectiveness (Fisher, P. B. et al., 2019). Tumour-infiltrating lymphocytes consist of all lymphocytic cell populations that have invaded the tumour tissue. Tumour-infiltrating lymphocytes have been caught in several solid tumours, including breast cancer, and are emerging as an important biomarker in predicting the efficacy and result of immunotherapy. In breast cancer, Tumour-infiltrating lymphocytes are comprised primarily of cytotoxic (CD8+) and helper T cells and a smaller proportion of B- and NK cells (Fisher, P. B. et al., 2019). Tumour-specific T cells are often present in the peripheral blood of cancer patients and infiltrate tumours, yet these T cells are generally unable to direct regression of bulky tumours.

One significant advance in the immunotherapeutic treatment of breast cancer is the success of adoptive T cell therapy, where autologous tumour-specific T cells are expanded and then reinfused into the cancer patient. Adoptive T cell therapy and tumour-infiltrating lymphocytes have emerged as one of the most potent therapies for metastatic melanoma, with a 50% response rate (Fisher, P. B. et al., 2019). While these methods have made strides in treatment, small tumour sizes or pretreatment with radiation or chemotherapy can render a tumour not optimal for the outgrowth of tumour-infiltrating lymphocytes because of the small size or destruction of the tumour-infiltrating lymphocytes (Fisher, P. B. et al., 2019). While innovative, immunotherapy using tumour infiltrating lymphocytes and adoptive T-cell therapy has limited success in breast cancer patients. Other dendritic cells based vaccination show promise in producing anti-tumour immunity. They are not enough to eliminate the self-antigen propitiated immune threshold.

Approaches applied in modern immunotherapy are based on complementation or stimulation of the immune system by employing compounds, such as lymphokines, which act upon cells of the immune system, vaccines, and in vitro-stimulated effector cells of the immune system antibodies (Schuster et al., 2006). The research directed by Coley discovered that the immune system could be stimulated to control tumour growth and, in some cases, destroy an existing solid tumour. Therefore if tumour cells are recognized in an immunogenic context, the immune system can attack (Schuster et al., 2006). Immunotherapy is a promising addition and eventually a possible alternative to the traditional invasive cancer treatment methods.

ADOPTIVE T-CELL TRANSFER THERAPY

From the 1940s to the 1960s, many researchers independently noticed a strange phenomenon. When they injected mice with oncogenic viruses—viruses that caused the mice to develop tumours—the immune systems of the mice would recognize the antigens from the virus on the tumour cells and destroy the tumours (Coulie et al., 2014). Initially, they assumed that the immune system only attacked the tumour because it was caused by a virus (Coulie et al., 2014). But, even if the tumours were induced with carcinogenic chemicals and lacked viral antigens, the immune systems of the mice still attacked the tumours (Coulie et al., 2014). These foundational studies were the first to show that T cells have the innate capability to attack tumour cells. From these studies, many new cancer therapies have been developed. Specifically, this chapter will focus on adoptive T cell transfer therapy.

Adoptive T cell transfer therapy refers to a type of cancer treatment where T cells are injected into the patient's bloodstream. These cells are called cytotoxic T cells: their role is to specifically bind to molecules on the surface of tumour cells called antigens. Once attached to the antigens on tumour cells, they lyse (or kill) them. There are two main types of adoptive T cell therapy, which differ based on the origin of the T cells: autologous or allogeneic. Autologous cells are taken from the patient, while allogeneic cells are harvested from a donor (June, 2007). However, while many researchers have investigated the first type of therapy, there is a much smaller body of research on the second.

For this reason, this chapter will mainly focus on autologous adoptive T cell transfer cell therapy, also called tumour-infiltrating lymphocyte (TIL) treatment. Three key areas will be covered:

1. The methodology and theory behind TIL therapy will be ad dressed.

2. Its strengths and limitations will be explored.

3. The chapter will finish by outlining various adaptations of traditional TIL therapy that have been engineered to address its limitations.

Tumour-infiltrating lymphocyte (TIL) therapy is the primary form of adoptive T cell therapy. In this form of therapy, cytotoxic T cells, which specifically target and kill tumour cells, are extracted from the patient's tumour. While these cells are theoretically capable of killing tumour cells, they cannot eradicate the tumour because they are insufficient in number. There are too many immunosuppressive cells within the tumour (Lee and Margolin, 2012). The rationale of TIL therapy is that if these cells are removed from the immunosuppressive environment of the tumour and allowed to replicate to large numbers before being injected into the patient, they will be able to eradicate the tumour (Lee and Margolin, 2012).

The procedure is as follows (Lee and Margolin, 2012). First, the tumour is harvested, and T cells from within the tumour are isolated and placed in media to allow them to grow and replicate. IL-2 is added, which causes the cells to reproduce very quickly, while the tumour cells adhered to them die or are killed by the T cells themselves. After two to four weeks, the T cells will be tested for their ability to destroy a sample of the patient's tumour cells. The cells which are the most reactive to the tumour cells will be isolated and once again placed in media to allow them to replicate as quickly as possible for the next two weeks. At this time, the T cells will be intravenously injected into the patient.

Frequently, for TIL therapy to be more successful, the patient must undergo lymphodepletion first (June, 2007). Lymphodepletion is when a patient undergoes chemotherapy or radiation therapy intending to deplete their immune system by killing white blood cells, also known as lymphocytes (June, 2007). Lymphodepletion kills the immunosuppressive cells which would normally prevent the TIL cells from replicating within the tumour and killing cancer cells (Lee and Margolin, 2012). Also, in the body, all the lymphocytes compete to bind IL-7 and IL-17, which cause the cells to grow and replicate (Lee and Margolin, 2012). Lymphodepletion decreases the number of total lymphocytes in the body, decreasing the competition for IL-7 and IL-15, meaning that more of the TIL cells will bind and therefore grow and replicate (Lee and Margolin, 2012).

So far, numerous clinical trials have supported the efficacy of TIL therapy for metastatic melanoma, i.e. patients whose melanoma has spread to other areas besides the original site of the tumour (Rohaan et al., 2018). For example, a clinical trial by Rosenberg and colleagues in 2011 found response rates of 49 to 72% of metastatic melanoma tumours, depending on the type of lymphodepletion regimen used before TIL therapy (Rosenberg et al., 2011). Amazingly, 20 of 93 patients showed complete regression of their cancers, and 19 of these individuals still showed complete reversal after three years (Rosenberg et al., 2011). Another clinical trial with metastatic melanoma patients by Radvanyi et al. (2012) found that 15 of 31 patients' tumours regressed partially, while 2 of these patients showed complete regression. 9 of the 15 patients' tumours did not progress (get larger) after 12 months (Radvanyi et al., 2012). A smaller study by Dudley et al. (2002) found that about half of metastatic melanoma patients showed tumour regression, although their sample size was only 13 patients.

While several studies show TIL therapy to be successful in melanoma, only a few are investigating its efficacy for other cancers. For instance, in 2012, Stevanović and colleagues found that 3 of 9 patients with metastatic cervical cancer showed tumour regression after being treated with TIL therapy. Of these three, one showed complete remission (Stevanović et al., 2012). Also, Lee et al. (2017) used TIL therapy on breast cancer cells *in vitro* (outside the body). They found that TIL cells were reactive to tumour cells. They also implanted breast cancer tumour tissue into mice, then treated them with TIL therapy. In this circumstance, too, the treatment proved effective. While these two studies show preliminary support for the efficacy of TIL therapy in cervical and breast cancers, Stevanović et al. (2015) is limited by small sample size, and Lee et al. (2017) performs only *in vitro* or animal research.

As discussed in the past two paragraphs, many studies support the usefulness of TIL therapy in abolishing tumours. Still, there are several limitations associated with this type of therapy. Over the rest of the chapter, the nature of these limitations and the ways in which TIL therapy has been adapted to overcome these limitations will be discussed.

One pressing limitation of TIL therapy is the time required to generate enough TIL cells for treatment. As previously mentioned, this process typically takes about 5 to 6 weeks (June, 2007). However, patients with rapidly progressing or particularly aggressive cancers may not be able to wait for the treatment to be ready (June, 2007). For this reason, a modified procedure termed the "Young TIL" protocol was developed by Dudley et al. (2010). The protocol for this method is similar to the traditional TIL method, except that it skips the selection step, where only cells that are highly reactive to the tumour cells are replicated (Dudley et al., 2010). Because the selection step is skipped, the TIL cells are less reactive to the tumour. Still, less time is required to generate a sufficiently large number to initiate therapy in the patient: the young TIL procedure requires only 25 days to generate enough TIL, whereas the traditional method requires about 45 (Lee and Margolin, 2012). As a result of a quicker generation time, TIL therapy is a feasible option for many patients (Lee and Margolin, 2012).

Moreover, cells that spend less time *in vitro* (outside the body) express higher CD27 and CD28 and have longer telomeres (Lee and Margolin, 2012). CD27 and CD28 expression are associated with the increased ability of T cells to replicate within the body. As T cells approach senescence, their CD27 and CD28 levels progressively drop, meaning that higher CD27 and CD28 are earlier in their life cycle (Larbi and Fulop, 2014). Similarly, longer telomeres are also associated with a T cell's ability to proliferate (Larbi and Fulop, 2014). Since TIL cells using the Young TIL protocol have higher CD27 and CD28 and longer telomeres, they should remain functional for a more extended period once injected into the body. Correspondingly, even when traditional TIL therapy is used, researchers have noted that longer telomeres and higher numbers of cells with CD28 and CD27 are associated with tumour regression (Rosenberg et al., 2011). Furthermore, in comparing traditional and young TIL therapies, cells from the young TIL protocol showed higher CD27 levels and longer telomeres than cells from the conventional protocol (Donia et al., 2011). TIL cells from both protocols showed similar reactivity to the tumour cells, highlighting that young TIL therapy shows promise as an equally effective therapy for individuals with rapidly progressing cancers (Donia et al., 2011).

Another critical limitation of TIL therapy is that some tumours are poorly antigenic (June, 2007). Some tumours may only express surface molecules that are the same as those described on normal cells, and some tumours may produce unique antigens but not a sufficient number to generate a T cell response (Coulie et al., 2014). In fact, because of the prevalence of poor antigenicity in tumours, only 30 to 40% of tumour specimens taken from patients will result in the successful generation of TIL (June, 2007). A new TIL therapy known as T cell receptor (TCR) gene therapy was developed to solve this problem. In this therapy, a T cell receptor specific to the tumour antigen is either isolated or designed (Wu et al., 2012). A particular type of virus capable of editing cells' genes is then used to insert the TCR gene into T cells from the human patient (Schmitt et al., 2009). Once this has occurred, the T cells can now express the TCR on their surfaces, use the TCR to bind tumour cells, and ultimately kill them.

Under normal circumstances, poorly antigenic tumours will not produce a T cell response. However, if TCR is inserted into the T cells, they can attack the tumour anyway. At first glance, TCR gene therapy appears a satisfying solution to traditional TIL therapy limitations, but there are several very limiting concerns with this new therapy. First, while TIL cells typically recognize several antigens present on tumour cells, TCR cells acknowledge only a single antigen (Wu et al., 2012). Tumour cells undergo genetic mutation quickly, which could allow a phenomenon known as immunoselection to occur (Wu et al., 2012). Some cells will randomly mutate not to have the antigens (Wu et al., 2012). Since only the cells with antigens are killed, soon the only cells remaining in the tumour are without the antigen (Wu et al., 2012). The TCR cells cannot recognize tumour cells without the antigen, and so the tumour continues to grow (Wu et al., 2012).

Another concerning limitation of TCR gene therapy is that it may result in severe side effects (Coulie et al., 2014). As previously mentioned, not all tumour antigens are tumour-specific; some of these antigens exist in normal cells. TCR is designed to be highly reactive to the antigen, so they are likely to attack antigens on normal body cells as well (Coulie et al., 2014). When they attack normal body cells, they can not only cause unpleasant side effects, but they can even cause the patient to die (Coulie et al., 2014). Another potentially lethal complication of TCR therapy is graft-versus-host-disease (GVHD), where the immune system attacks the injected TCR cells (Bendle et al., 2010). When the immune system targets TCR cells, it releases large amounts of inflammatory proteins called cytokines (Bendle et al., 2010). This "cytokine storm" can be highly damaging or even lethal to patients (Bendle et al., 2010). Even if GVHD were less dangerous, it also presents another problem: it destroys the TCR cells, so the tumour remains intact (Bendle et al., 2010).

A final limitation of TCR gene therapy is that they can only attack antigens under specific circumstances. TCR cells can only attack tumour cells if the antigen is present on the tumour cell's surface attached to a protein of the immune system known as MHC I (Wu et al., 2012). However, because cancer occurs partially due to a failure of the immune system, antigens are not always present attached to MHC I molecules, meaning that TCR cells would not be able to recognize them to kill the tumour cell (Wu et al., 2012). This particular limitation considerably restricts the use of TCR therapy, and so a variation of TCR gene therapy has been developed, known as chimeric antigen receptor (CAR) therapy.

Chimeric antigen receptors are very similar to TCRs in that they, too, are specifically engineered to recognize a tumour antigen (June and Sadelain, 2018). Like TCRs, they are then inserted into T cells using special viruses which transfer genetic information (June and Sadelain, 2018). Yet, unlike TCRs, CARs recognize antigens even when they are not bound to MHC I proteins, making CAR gene therapy applicable to many more tumours and patients than TCR gene therapy (June and Sadelain, 2018). The technology behind CAR therapy is incredible. CARs contain two regions: the binding and signalling sections (Ramos and Dotti, 2011). The binding section is designed to bind very tightly to the tumour cell antigen (Ramos and Dotti, 2011). Because the binding section is intended to bind the antigen and not the MHC I protein (as in TCR), MHC I is not required for CAR therapy to work. However, the signalling portion is essentially the same as a normal T cell receptor to trigger tumour cell death as usual (Ramos and Dotti, 2011).

Besides being applicable to many clinical situations, CAR gene therapy holds a few more advantages over TCR gene therapy. As previously mentioned, TCR therapy requires antigens to be attached to MHC I. However, this is not the only factor limiting when TCR cells can attack tumour cells. TCRs can only recognize protein antigens, while CARs can recognize any molecule (Ramos and Dotti, 2011). Considering that cells are often covered in glycoproteins and carbohydrates, identifying these molecules provides a considerable advantage. Moreover, CAR therapy confers a lower risk of GVHD than TCR therapy due to differences in the structure of the two receptors (Ramos and Dotti, 2011). Conversely, CAR therapy shares an important limitation with TCR therapy: immunoselection, a phenomenon where tumours mutate to no longer have the antigen recognized by TCR and CAR cells (Majzer and Mackall, 2018). Another serious disadvantage of CAR therapy is that it is associated with serious toxicities to both the nervous and immune systems (Mohanty, 2019).

Over the course of this chapter, an initial type of adoptive T cell therapy—TIL therapy—was explored in detail. Following a discussion of its limitations, two adapted forms of TIL were introduced: TCR and CAR gene therapies. TCR gene therapy was introduced to combat the poor antigenicity of tumours and/or the failure of the immune system to recognize tumour cells as a threat. CAR gene therapy, in turn, was developed in response to the limitations of TCR, in that TCR cells can only recognize antigens bound to MHC I proteins. Evidently, over the evolution of TIL therapy, many advances have been made. However, there are still many limitations that need to be overcome. I personally am very excited to see what this field has in store for us in the future: perhaps T cells engineered to persist in the body or even a cure for GVHD.

IMMUNE CHECKPOINT THERAPY

T lymphocytes (also referred to as T cells) play a vital role in the immuno-surveillance of cancer; they are immune cells that work alongside immune checkpoints to ensure foreign antigens or infected cells are eradicated (Jenkins et al., 2018). As such, T cells aid in cancer treatment as they can recognize, infiltrate and destroy any host cancerous tumour cells by identifying a self-antigen. The process of recognizing cancerous cells in the immune system is through memory. Once the immune system has encountered a foreign object, the antigen specificity is acquired, allowing the T cells to become more diverse and carry the new information to destroy any other cells with the same antigen specificity (Sharma et al., 2021).

Concerns emerge when the immune checkpoints interfere with cancer treatment by inducing adverse T cell regulatory pathways by immune checkpoints forming bonds with their partner proteins. Essentially, turning the immune cells "off" from eradicating the cancerous cells. Negative protein regulators of anti-T cell pathways are CTLA-4, PD-1, and PD-L1, promoting anti-tumour eradication (Jenkins et al., 2018). This is where Immune Checkpoint Therapies (ICT) is implemented to reverse this process by decreasing and ultimately stopping the occurrence of proteins CTLA-4, PD-1, and PD-L1 from promoting tumour eradication once more. Immune Checkpoint Therapy does this through checkpoint inhibitors that preclude the proteins CTLA-4, PD-1, and PD-L1 from forming a bond with their partner proteins, thus putting a stop to the "off" signal in T cells (Jenkins et al., 2018). Immune Checkpoint Therapy provides blockages to immune checkpoints so that the positive effector regulatory immune pathway occurs, whereas the adverse path with antitumour T cells are shut off.

As there have been many scientific advances in T cell immunobiology, Immune Checkpoint Therapy is the most instrumental in which immune checkpoint blockade can be administered and regulated. Immune Checkpoint Therapy is distributed in the form of an immunotherapy drug. Different drugs and medications have differing effects on the three protein checkpoint inhibitors CTLA-4, PD-1, and PD-L1 and have other side effects.

The drug Ipilimumab (Yervoy) effectively diminishes the CTLA-4 protein and is administered intravenously for ninety-minute regimen doses every three weeks (Webster, 2014). Ipilimumab is a monoclonal antibody (man-made antibody) that attaches to the CTLA-4 protein and creates a blockade from it to bind to its partner protein, making the adverse T cell feedback pathway. Clinically, Ipilimumab has shown the most promise in aiding those with skin (with an emphasis on melanoma), colorectal, renal, lung, and hepatocellular (a form of the liver) cancer (Ruan et al., 2019).

The drugs pembrolizumab (Keytruda), Nivolumab (Opdivo), and cemiplimab (Libtayo) target the anti-T cell protein PD-1 and are administered intravenously. They are issued for 30 minutes every three weeks, 60 minutes every two weeks, and 30 minutes every three weeks, respectively (Webster, 2014). These monoclonal antibodies attach themselves to the PD-1 protein on the surface of immune cells, allowing T cells to continue to destroy cancerous tumour cells in the body. Types of cancers these drugs treat most effectively include bladder, renal pelvis, ureter (urethra), skin (with an emphasis on melanoma) cancer (Ruan et al., 2019).

The drugs Atezolizumab (Tecentriq), Avelumab (Bavencio), and Durvalumab (Imfinzi) are vital in blockading the PD-L1 protein and is administered intravenously for 30-60 minutes every three weeks, 60 minutes every two weeks, and 60 minutes every four weeks, respectively (Webster, 2014). These drugs attack the PD-L1 negative anti-T cell pathway regulation by binding to the protein to create a blockage, allowing the immune system T cells to eradicate the cancerous tumour cells. Types of cancers that these drugs have the most efficient outcomes include breast (emphasis on triple-negative breast cancer), lung (focus on small cell lung cancer), bladder, urinary, and liver cancer (Ruan et al., 2019).

Although Immune Checkpoint Therapy drugs have significant effects in treating various forms of cancer through checkpoint inhibitors like any medication prescribed, some possible side effects can negatively affect the patient. The immune checkpoint inhibitors cause some adverse effects named immune-related adverse events (irAEs). The different combinations of drugs and treatment plans on top of individual patients have differing effects and levels. Fatal or near-death incidents occur approximately 0.3-1.3% of the time, and usually, very early on, physicians can adjust the treatment plan based on adverse prognosis effects (Martins et al., 2019). This rate increases with immune checkpoint therapy combined with allogeneic hematopoietic treatment and decreases with immune checkpoint therapy combined with platinum-doublet chemotherapy or targeted therapy (examples include tyrosine kinase inhibitors or vascular endothelial growth factor targeted agents). In a clinical study done in 2018 by Martins et al., the drug Ipilimumab that provides antibodies for the protein CTLA-4 has the highest fatalities in patients with irAE; 70% or 135 out of 193 patients. On the contrary, the drugs administered for anti-PD-1 and anti-PD-L1 have fewer adverse side effects, including 35% or 115 out of 333 getting pneumonitis, 22% or 75 out of 333 getting hepatitis, and 15% or 50 out of 333 having neurotoxic symptoms (Martins et al., 2019). The clinical studies proved that combination therapies attributed to the most deaths instead of targeted therapies, including 37% or 32 out of 87 patients getting colitis and 25% or 22 out of 87 patients having myocarditis (Martins et al., 2019).

Less adverse but more common and minor side effects occur in patients as well. These effects differ based on the drug, dosage, and patient. Overall risks include rash, diarrhea, fatigue, rashes, skin inflammation/irritation, skin colour changes, muscle weakness/numbness, and difficulties breathing regularly (Hargadon et al., 2018). Immune checkpoint inhibitors epidemiology states that neurological conditions can also arise alongside physical side effects, but these are extremely rare. When neurological disorders occur, physicians are prompted to complete biopsy and tests, which will aid them in altering the treatment plan to meet the patient's needs for the most optimal cancer prognosis. Neurological autoimmune diseases and conditions exhibit themselves around two to twelve weeks after treatment is given (Sharma et al., 2021). Illnesses that arise in patients include inflammatory myopathies, myasthenia gravis, acute and chronic demyelinating polyradiculoneuropathies, vasculitic neuropathies, isolated cranial neuropathies, aseptic meningitis, autoimmune encephalitis, multiple sclerosis and hypophysitis (Hargadon et al., 2018).

The anti-CTLA-4 protein drug Ipilimumab side effects comprise feeling tired, diarrhea, nausea, itching, rash, vomiting, headache, weight loss, fever, decreased appetite, and difficulty falling or staying asleep (Ruan et al., 2019). The anti-PD-1 protein drugs Pembrolizumab (Keytruda), Nivolumab (Opdivo), and Cemiplimab (Libtayo) side effects consist of anemia, fatigue, hyperglycemia, hyponatremia, hypoalbuminemia, itching, cough, and nausea (Webster, 2014). The anti-PD-L1 protein drugs Atezolizumab (Tecentriq), Avelumab (Bavencio), and Durvalumab (Imfinzi) side effects include black stools, bladder pain, face swelling, body aches or pain, burning/painful urination, difficulty breathing, ear congestion, tiredness and weakness (Ruan et al., 2019).

Although Immune Checkpoint Therapy (ICT) is highly effective for some patients, in others, no such responses are seen. Through patient studies and clinical workups, it has been found that Immune Checkpoint Therapy works better in some cancers as opposed to others. Immune checkpoint therapy has been approved to be effective in helping treat patients with breast, bladder, cervical, colon, liver, renal, skin, stomach, rectal, and head/neck cancers. In addition, numerous clinical studies have been conducted on the basis of whether checkpoint inhibitors are effective in improving the prognosis of these various forms of cancers.

Despite the fact that pancreatic cancer is considered a rare form as it accounts for 3% of all cancers, it has the highest mortality rate. A study conducted by Johansson et al., in 2016 explored many different treatment combinations and drug therapies to track the success rate of the varying checkpoint inhibitors on patients with pancreatic cancer. Overall, the results suggest that although Immune Checkpoint Therapy is not a cure, it allows patients more time and effectively improves the prognosis of the disease. The drug Ipilimumab used in combination with other therapies increased survival by 5.7 months, but the drug Ipilimumab alone resulted in a 3.6-month increase in patient's lives (Johansson et al., 2016). The disease was stabilized (no unfavourable prognosis) in very few patients, around 5-10% when treated with 10mg/kg of Ipilimumab (Johansson et al., 2016). Partial positive responses and stabilization of the disease were seen in even fewer patients when treated with 15mg/kg of drugs Durvalumab and Tremelimumab. Although little positive prognosis was shown, the survival rate of patients with this therapy overall increased by 7.4 months (Johansson et al., 2016). Due to a small number of participants being a limitation of the studies conducted, the researchers prompt for a larger-scale clinical trial to be done, but currently, the checkpoint inhibitors seem to be a growing vitality in pancreatic cancer treatment.

Liver cancer is the sixth most common form of cancer, and it is the second most common cause of cancer-related deaths. A clinical trial completed in 2018 by Xu et al., took previous research done on Immune Checkpoint Therapy with small cell lung cancer, renal cell carcinoma, melanoma, lymphoma, and urothelial bladder cancer and altered the dosages of immune checkpoint drug inhibitors to affect liver cancer patients positively. The immune checkpoint drugs that are being used in this study include Nivolumab, Pembrolizumab, and Ipilimumab. The success rate of a 3 mg/kg dose of Nivolumab is 20% in the beginning, and after a while, it goes down to 15%, as the body gets used to such (Xu et al., 2018). The data from combined drug therapies have a 17% success rate in aiding to treat cholangiocarcinoma. Researchers also found through analysis that immune checkpoint inhibitors may fail to work on certain patients as their prospective cancers have mutations resulting from the immunogenicity of the drugs, the expression of the drugs on the tumour cells, and immune T cell defects (Xu et al., 2018).

Breast cancer is the most common type of cancer in women worldwide, but it can happen in both women and men. A research study in 2017 by Solinas et al. explored the performance of drugs that fight against the checkpoint inhibitors PD-1 and PD-L1. Thirty-two patients were given the drug Pembrolizumab, which resulted in a favourable prognosis difference in around 58% of individuals (Solinas et al., 2017). More long-term differences have been seen in about 46.9% of patients, as 22% had increased life expectancy after two years. The tumours in those participating in the clinical trial decreased in 62% of patients, and 58% reduced new tumour cells (Solinas et al., 2017). Twenty-five participants treated with an extra high dosage of anti-PD-L1 drugs had maintained a favourable prognosis after 7.3 months. The drug Atezolizumab used in monotherapy was given to 115 participants, where 44.4% had positive outcomes on the expression of tumour infiltrating immune cells, even after twenty-eight weeks (Solinas et al., 2017).

Melanoma is a form of skin cancer known to be the fastest spreading form of cancer worldwide. Khair et al. performed a clinical research trial in 2019 to test various drug effects on patients with advanced beginner melanoma. Anti-PD-1 monoclonal antibody drugs Ipilimumab, Nivolumab, and Pembrolizumab were all implemented. Nivolumab increases patient survival rate by 8.9 months and 72.9% positive outcomes after six months of treatment (Khair et al., 2019). Advanced melanoma patients were unresponsive to Ipilimumab treatments, but 28% had a positive prognosis after Nivolumab treatments (Khair et al., 2019). The patients that received combined Ipilimumab and Nivolumab treatments exhibited the most promising outcomes, as survival rates after one year of treatment were the highest between all of the groups. On the contrary, this also came with the highest amount of adverse side effects in those that the combination therapy did not work (Khair et al., 2019).

Lung cancer is the most common type of cancer worldwide, and it is also the leading cause of cancer death for both men and women in America. The study in 2014 by Dr. Creelan looks at the anti-inhibitory protein drug effects alongside lung cancer and the killer immunoglobulin receptor (KIR). Trial results indicated that monoclonal antibodies of Nivolumab had the capability of reducing negative tumour rates by 20 to 25% in patients with lung cancer (Creelan, 2014). After data analysis, it was also found that a combination of anti-CTLA-4, anti-PD-1, and anti-PD-L1 blockade drugs increase positive tumour reduction responses (Creelan, 2014). This research concludes that combination drug therapies are most effective for helping eradicate cancerous tumour cells in epithelial lung cancer.

Much progress, research, and advancements have been made regarding Immune Checkpoint Therapy, but that does not mean everything that can be known has been as of now. In the future, more research and studies should be dedicated to adjusting the anti-protein drugs to create more suitable treatment therapies. Many adverse side effects are seen in some patients who intravenously intake the anti-CTLA-4, anti-PD-1, and anti-PD-L1 drugs. To reduce and eradicate the rate of such, further testing is essential so that the drugs only have positive outcomes for those struggling with cancer instead of adding more issues to their prognosis. Additionally, further research is critical with more cancers than the Ministry of Health already approves regarding implementing anti-protein drugs to specific cancer treatment plans. For example, the effects on such immune checkpoint inhibitory drugs have not yet been researched or tested with prostate, brain, bronchial, gallbladder, ovarian, gastric, thyroid, and more various forms of cancer. Other specific challenges regarding Immune Checkpoint Therapy are further understanding the pathways of resistance, increasing patient selection regarding treatment plans, and finding new therapeutic combinations for maximum success (Acevedo et al., 2018).

T lymphocytes (also referred to as T cells) are a fundamental part of cancer treatment as T cells are a part of the immune system that can infiltrate and eradicate cancerous cells. Immune cell inhibitors that come in the form of CTLA-4, PD-1, and PD-L1 proteins block T cells from doing their job to destroy cancerous tumour cells, ultimately creating an adverse regulatory pathway damaging to a patient's cancer prognosis. Immune Checkpoint Therapy becomes essential to reverse these effects and block the immune cell inhibitors from turning the T cells "off." Immune Checkpoint Therapy is administered intravenously through varying drugs that blockade the three anti-positive regulatory pathway proteins. The drug Ipilimumab (Yervoy) effectively diminishes the CTLA-4 protein, and side effects include feeling tired, diarrhea, nausea, itching, rash, vomiting, headache, weight loss, fever, decreased appetite, and difficulty falling or staying asleep. The drugs Pembrolizumab (Keytruda), Nivolumab (Opdivo), and Cemiplimab (Libtayo) target the anti-T cell protein PD-1, and side effects consist of anemia, fatigue, hyperglycemia, hyponatremia, hypoalbuminemia, itching, cough, and nausea. The drugs Atezolizumab (Tecentriq), Avelumab (Bavencio), and Durvalumab (Imfinzi) blockade the PD-L1 protein and side effects include black stools, bladder pain, face swelling, body aches or pain, burning/painful urination, difficulty breathing, ear congestion, tiredness and weakness. More adverse side effects of immune checkpoint inhibitors include pneumonitis, hepatitis, colitis, myocarditis, myasthenia gravis, acute/chronic demyelinating polyradiculoneuropathies, vasculitic neuropathies, isolated cranial neuropathies, aseptic meningitis, autoimmune encephalitis, multiple sclerosis and hypophysitis. The various forms of cancer that Immune Checkpoint Therapy aids in the prognosis of treatment are breast, bladder, pancreatic, cervical, colon, liver, lung, renal, skin (emphasis on melanoma), stomach, rectal, head, neck, and urinary cancers. Thus, Immune Checkpoint Therapy is essential in providing patients undergoing cancer treatments with positive prognosis reports due to the immune checkpoint inhibitors administered through intravenous drugs to increase patient survival.

THE PROMISE OF CANCER VACCINES

The concept of a vaccine for various cancers has long been a source of hope and excitement for both researchers looking to innovate the way cancer is treated, and also the cancer patient with their friends and family. There have been two rises in the popularity of studying the immunogenicity of cancer and its potential for new treatment pathways. One of these resulted in widespread disillusionment and disappointment, the other with more fruitful discoveries which seem to be happening all around us at the present time from studies and clinical trials all around the world. Many vaccines exist in the medical field and are constantly being researched to prevent disease. The challenge presented with developing a vaccine for cancer versus a vaccine for an infectious disease is that most of the latter kind of vaccines are prophylactic, meaning they prevent a disease from developing. Two preventive cancer vaccines already exist. First, the "human papillomavirus (HPV) vaccine prevents infection, where chronic HPV is a risk factor for the development of cervical cancer." (Zhou et al., 2015). This HPV vaccine is routinely administered to young girls as a normal part of a child's recommended vaccinations. The second is a vaccine to prevent infection by hepatitis B virus (HBV), which has a "high risk of progression to cirrhosis and hepatocellular carcinoma" (Zhou et al., 2015).

In comparison, a vaccine to treat cancer would primarily need to be therapeutic. It would need to target and eradicate cancerous cells that already exist in the body and evade the body's dysfunctional immune system which has allowed the growth of a tumour. When the immunogenicity of cancer (meaning the extent to which the foreign object will provoke an immune response of some kind in the body) was realized, it was observed in cancer patients with tumour progression that the secretion of immunosuppressive factors and downregulation of the ways the immune system can recognize an antigen as nonself occur.

At this point in time, as Gilboa (2004) wrote, "the question of cancer vaccination, therefore, [was] not 'if' but 'how.'"

To solve this 'how' question, various obstacles must be overcome. Similar to how infectious disease vaccines work, to elicit an immune response against a cancerous tumour, the appropriate antigen must be presented to a naive T cell by specialized cells called antigen-presenting cells (APCs). These APCs regulate immunity by taking up antigens from the vaccine, showing them to and bring about differentiation of naive T cells into memory and effector T cells (Gilboa, 2004). Some difficulty arises around using this bodily procedure to the advantage of the vaccine, specifically which antigen is selected. According to Shibata et al., the best properties for the chosen antigen to have in an ideal situation are "cancer cell-specific expression, high immunogenicity and, ideally, a cancer cell-specific functional dependency" (2020). They cite two possible avenues of development: tumour-associated antigens and tumour-specific antigens. Tumour-associated antigens are strongly expressed in cancer cells and make a good target for T cells. However, they are also retained weakly in normal tissues. With this comes a "possibility of inducing autoimmune toxicity in normal tissues, such as colitis, hepatitis, or rapid respiratory failure" (Shibata et al., 2020). An example of a cancer-associated antigen in a clinical trial testing its efficacy in treating patients with solid tumours is telomerase (hTERT). "hTERT functions to support cancer cell growth and survival, most directly by maintaining telomeres to support cancer cell immortality," writes Slingluff (2019). In mouse models, vaccination against hTERT increased infiltration of T cells into B16 melanomas, but human trials still need to be performed.

Tumour-specific antigens, or neoantigens, are not found in non-cancerous cells. The immune system would recognize these antigens as nonself and "are less likely to induce autoimmunity compared to [tumour-associated antigens]" (Shibata et al., 2020). A promising new avenue for treatment for head and neck squamous cell carcinoma comes from research around antigens specific to HPV-related cancers such as the oncoproteins E6 and E7. Oncoproteins have the ability to transform a cell into a tumour if they are introduced. Tumour cells are genetically unstable because of the repeated mutations of DNA that accumulate as cancer grows. These mutations can be classified into two groups: driver mutations which "mainly contribute to cancer development," and passenger mutations that are not involved with the disease's further activity or progression (Shibata et al., 2020). Similarly to the way, the driver of the car is the only one with the influence over the speed and direction, and the passenger does not. Groups are looking into neoantigens from driver mutations shared among patients and those looking for combinations of passenger mutations; however, it is reportedly difficult to predict these tumour-specific antigens. To address this issue, Shibata et al. share the growing calls for "targeted sequencing of cancer-related gene mutations… and building an inventory of shared neoantigen peptide libraries of common solid tumours" (2020). These databases of neoantigens have "reduced the time from prediction to patient vaccination," something that is so very crucial in progressive and challenging deadly diseases (Shibata et al., 2020).

The term vaccination platform refers to the mechanism by which the antigen is delivered to the antigen-presenting cells. It can be thought of as the mode of transportation the vaccine uses to get the antigen to the environment in which the tumour is. There are three main ways to categorize these platforms, all of which are seeing considerable research. The first is peptide vaccines. Peptides are short chains of amino acids; short peptides have under eleven, and longer peptides have more. This is a popular vaccine platform, with many clinical trials completed and the next steps being considered. Short peptides "do not require processing by APCs," offering an advantage to longer peptide chains which must be taken up and processed by antigen-presenting cells (Shibata et al., 2020). While this ability to skip a step may seem appealing, clinical trials have found a risk of dysfunction in the immune system if short peptide chains stimulate T cells without the presence of other stimulating factors or adjuvants. Antigen-presenting cells with long peptide chain-derived antigens "can activate CTL or helper T cells without inducing energy by transmitting signals via both T cell receptors (TCRs) and costimulatory molecules," avoiding the problem altogether (Igarashi & Sasada, 2020). As such, the development of long peptide vaccines is being researched and pursued.

Nucleic acid-based vaccines have a few advantages over other vaccine platforms in that they will "allow for the delivery of multiple antigens covering various... somatic tumour mutations, eliciting both humoral and cell-mediated immune response" (Miao et al., 2021). The nucleic acids can hold the genetic code for the production of multiple antigens in one vaccine. While peptide vaccines are time and labour intensive to produce, nucleic acid vaccines are "inexpensive and can be synthesized stably" (Igarashi & Sasada, 2020). Another advantage that nucleic acid-based vaccines have over peptides is that the genetic code can often be carried within a viral vector. The nucleic acids will be taken into the cells much more efficiently as the immune system recognizes the virus used as non-self. Igarashi and Sasada (2020) warn that "the disadvantage of viral vectors is that repeated administration might be difficult due to the induction of antiviral immune responses." There are two forms the nucleic acids may take, DNA and RNA. Each has advantages and disadvantages, but it seems like RNA holds the most promise for researchers because, unlike DNA it does "not need to penetrate the nuclear membrane and can function when they are delivered to the cytoplasm of APCs" (Shibata et al., 2020). Messenger RNA platforms have been "experiencing a considerable burst in preclinical and clinical research," with "over twenty mRNA-based immunotherapies have entered clinical trials with some promising outcomes in solid tumour treatments" (Miao et al., 2021). There have been exciting innovations with mRNA-based vaccines that are not related to cancer, namely the FDA approval of Pfizer-BioNTech and Moderna COVID-19 vaccines. This rise in interest in mRNA vaccine technology will undoubtedly lead to innovations and research for both infectious diseases and cancer mRNA-based vaccines. A specific type of mRNA is being explored that will maximize the vaccine's effect in terms of the length of time and magnitude of the production of antigens. Self-amplifying mRNA (SAM) originates from viruses that carry single-stranded mRNA. It consists of two main regions or open reading frames, one that encodes the antigen sequence and the other that encodes proteins and structures that will amplify the mRNA and the immune response to the growing number of antigens. The strand has been modified so that the genes which encode the viral particles and structures are "replaced with gene[s] encoding the antigen(s) of interest" (Miao et al., 2021). While the genetic instructions for the viral infectious parts are removed from the RNA strand, the instructions for the replication machinery remain and enable the RNA to be amplified within the cytoplasm of a cell. As discussed before, the challenge is using a viral vector lies in finding the tolerable viral burden and toxicities for people with cancer who already have a compromised immune system, and the potential for "pre-existing immunity to many of the viral backbones that are currently deemed safe in humans" (Bullock, 2021) affecting the efficacy of the therapy. The informative paper summarizing the current state of mRNA vaccines for cancer written by Miao et al. states that a "64-fold less dose of SAM achieved the equivalent immunity to the non-replicating mRNA" (2021). They also cite the superiority of mRNA-based vaccines as three-fold: the ability to encode more than a particular antigen; the ease of integration into the cell as well as the high degradability of mRNA by RNases compared to DNA, reducing the risk of mutations due to the integration of the nucleic acid into the cell's genes or the toxicity of built-up mRNA; and its ability to be synthesized rapidly and in a cost-efficient, scalable manner.

The third vaccination platform is certainly worth discussion as well. Cell-based vaccines involve the use of the individual patient's cancer cells. Irradiated cells from the tumour of the cancer patient are administered via vaccine along with an adjuvant, similarly to how peptide-based vaccines work. The adjuvant is able to "provide an inflammatory context for antigen presentation," meaning the T cells are being stimulated while being provided with the irradiated tumour cell which has, potentially, many antigens which could be targeted (Bullock, 2021). Igarashi and Sasada (2020) cite this approach being tested with many different types of cancers: colorectal cancer, lung cancer, renal cell carcinoma, prostate cancer, and melanoma. They go on to detail how cells may be genetically modified so that they have the capabilities of producing cytokines, signalling proteins that can facilitate inflammation, as well as a granulocyte-macrophage colony-stimulating factor (GM-CSF) which also act as cytokines that stimulate the production of granulocytes and monocytes. GVAX is a vaccine for cancer that uses genetically modified cancer cells that secrete granulocyte-macrophage colony-stimulating factor after a patient goes through radiation treatment. The purpose of the vaccine is to stop the uncontrollable growth of the tumour, thereby extending the life of the individual. Early clinical trials in phases one and two have found good results in non-small-cell lung carcinoma, "however, no effects have been seen in phase [three] clinical trials for prostate cancer" (Igarashi & Sasada, 2020).

Another cell-based avenue that is being explored is the possibility of using dendritic cells (DCs) as the vehicle for "a variety of antigens, including tumour cells, tumour-derived proteins or peptides, and DNA/RNA" (Igarashi & Sasada, 2020). Bullock (2021) describes the role of these cells in the body; dendritic cells are most often found in places that are likely to see exposure to the environment, including lungs, digestive tract, and the skin. When a cancer cell dies, sometimes due to nutrient deprivation, they get engulfed by DCs or other antigen-presenting cells. They are able not only to initiate the phagocytosis of the dying cancer cell and stimulate T cell activation, but they are also able to sense when there is something strange about its environment because of receptors on the cell's surface that recognize the signals that are released by a dying cell. The signals as a whole are referred to as "damage-associated molecular patterns (DAMPs)" (Bullock, 2021). Dendritic cells have an important job to play in the world of immunotherapeutics because they are able to "absorb and express tumour-associated antigens" (Xu et al., 2020). According to Miao et al., "DC-based mRNA vaccine therapies... account for [the] majority of mRNA cancer vaccines in clinical trials" (2021). A vaccine called Stipuleucel-T is developed using autologous cells, meaning cells from the body of the patient, and loaded up with prostatic acid phosphatase (PAP) and GM-CSF. PAP is specific to prostate cancer, and the Stipuleucel-T is an emerging "immunotherapy for castration-resistant prostate cancer" (Zhou et al., 2015).

Vaccines are also seeing breakthroughs in the therapeutic treatment of cancer through their combined effects with other more traditional cancer treatments. Traditional treatment avenues include radiotherapy which uses targeted and high dose radiation to shrink or kill tumour cells, chemotherapy which uses potent chemicals to stop the progression of the disease, and surgery which involves the removal of tumour tissue by a surgeon. According to Zhou et al., the novel immunotherapy treatments have "demonstrated the complementary role to traditional cancer treatments" (2015). A previously discussed form of cancer vaccine combined with radiation therapy in animal studies "significantly prolonged the overall survival of the animals" and showed "significant therapeutic efficacy... in the management of established tumours" (Zhou et al., 2015). In addition to this, the GVAX treatment also discussed earlier has been used in combination with radiation in patients with advanced pancreatic cancer and has shown promising results in several phases two trials.

Traditional methods of cancer treatments are not ideal. Although chemotherapy and radiotherapy are widely considered "the most important and effective therapeutic strategies for treating cancer," they also can "cause adverse reactions, drug resistance and long-term complications" (Xu et al., 2020). If we have known or encountered a cancer patient undergoing radiation or chemotherapy, we can speak to the obvious physical effects these treatments can have on an already struggling body. In media like television and movies, patients with cancer are run-down, have often lost their hair and are an unhealthy weight, just to name a few commonly seen cancer treatment side effects. In my own life, my grandmother battled breast cancer for eighteen years and went through many bouts of chemotherapy. After these chemicals entered her body, their toxic nature took a toll on her body. She lost her hair, her energy, and eventually her life when cancer came back. This is not an uncommon story around cancer, as it is globally the leading cause of death. With an expected "18 million new cancer cases and 9 million cancer deaths" each year, it is hard not to see the urgency in which we need to revolutionize our treatment of cancer (Xu et al., 2020).

EMERGING CANCER IMMUNOTHERAPETICS

Cancer immunotherapy techniques are proving to be practical tools in the fight against the disease. Checkpoint inhibitors' effectiveness in treating metastatic melanoma and adoptive T-cell therapy, with chimeric antigen receptor T cells treats B-cell–derived leukemias and lymphomas, which are only two examples of advances that are reshaping clinical cancer treatment (Zhou et al., 2015). These changes result from extensive research into the complex and interconnected cellular and molecular processes that regulate immune responses over several years (Zhou et al., 2015). The discovery of cancer mutation-encoded neoantigens, advancements in vaccine production, advancement in cellular therapy delivery, and remarkable achievements in biotechnology are all promising developments (Zhou et al., 2015).

As a result, cancer care is undergoing a dramatic transition, with traditional cancer therapies combined with immunotherapeutic agents. Many clinical studies are currently underway to evaluate the possible synergistic effects of treatments that combine immunotherapy and other therapies (Xu et al., 2020). There's still a lot to understand about product collection, distribution, and quality control, and off-target effects of immunotherapy used alone or in combination. Human tumours have developed various escape mechanisms from the host immune system, which remains an obstacle to success. The efforts to decipher the laws of immune cell dysfunction, cancer-related local, and systemic immune suppression yield new insights and ignite interest in novel therapeutic approaches. It could be possible in the future to adapt immunotherapy to the specific needs of each cancer patient. The use of new immune biomarkers and the ability to evaluate therapy responses by noninvasive testing have the potential to enhance cancer detection and prognosis in the early stages (Xu et al., 2020). Individualized immunotherapy focused on genetic, molecular, and immune profiling is a theoretically attainable target throughout the future. The current excitement for immunotherapy is justified because of many existing opportunities for harnessing the immune system to treat cancer (Xu et al., 2020).

"Various types of cancer immunotherapy were widely used in the 17th and 18th centuries... Septic dressings enclosing ulcerative tumours were used to treat cancer in the 18th and 19th centuries" (Gardner et al., 2012). Surgical wounds were left open to allow infection to spread, and purulent sores were purposefully developed (Gardner et al., 2012). In 1891, William Coley inoculated patients with inoperable tumours, resulting in one of the most well-known effects of microorganisms on cancer (Gardner et al., 2012). Coley thoroughly reviewed the literature available at that time and found 38 reports of cancer patients with accidental or iatrogenic feverish erysipelas. In 12 patients, the sarcoma or carcinoma had wholly disappeared; the others had substantially improved. Coley decided to attempt the therapeutic use of iatrogenic erysipelas Coley developed a toxin that contained heat-killed bacteria (Gardner et al., 2012). Until 1963, this treatment was used for the treatment of sarcoma (Gardner et al., 2012). 51.9% of patients with inoperable soft-tissue sarcomas showed complete tumour regression and survived for more than five years, and 21.2% of the patients had no clinical evidence of tumour at least 20 years after this treatment (Gardner et al., 2012). In cancer treatment, they aid cancer antigen targeting (Gardner et al., 2012). The only approved cellular cancer therapy based on dendritic cells is sepulture-T. One method of inducing dendritic cells to present tumour antigens is by vaccination with autologous tumour lysates or short peptides (Gardner et al., 2012). These peptides are often given in combination with adjuvants to increase the immune and antitumour responses. Other adjuvants include proteins or other chemicals that attract and activate dendritic cells, such as granulocyte-macrophage colony-stimulating factor. The most common source of antigens used for dendritic cell vaccine in Glioblastoma as an aggressive brain tumour were whole tumour lysate, CMV antigen RNA and tumour-associated peptides like EGFRAII (Gardner et al., 2012).

Clinical trials in cancer immunotherapy are essential for introducing new and potentially life-saving therapies to more patients with more forms of cancer. They may provide the best hope for those who are currently battling the disease. As clinical science advances, immunotherapy is becoming more widely available in clinical trials for early-stage cancers or as a first-line treatment choice (Igarashi & Sasada, 2020). On the other hand, many patients are unaware of recent immunotherapy breakthroughs and the increasing number of opportunities to engage in new cancer clinical trials. Patients will find it difficult to find cancer clinical trials that are suitable for them without this knowledge (Igarashi & Sasada, 2020).

Immunotherapy is a cutting-edge field of science that uses the body's immune system to combat cancer cells. Therapeutic antibodies (e.g., monoclonal antibodies, antibody-drug conjugates, and bispecific antibodies), checkpoint inhibitors (e.g., PD-1/PD-L1 inhibitors), adoptive cell therapies (e.g., CAR-T), and TCR therapies are all examples of these therapies (Lee and Margolin, 2012). One of the many problems that scientists face today is developing successful agents in patients with different forms of cancer. To include customized genetically engineered cells for novel cellular therapy and immunotherapy. Cell-based assay development to evaluate the efficacy, potency, & mechanism of action of candidate therapies.

- Expression of patient-specific or modified T cell receptors (TCRs) or CARs of interest using a modular "landing pad" cassette
- Tumour-associated antigen knockout or overexpression cell lines
- Checkpoint inhibitor knockout or overexpression cell lines
- Development of CAR-expression viral production cell lines
- Genome editing in primary immune cell lines

Engineered cell lines to evaluate cell or gene therapy(s) of interest (research use only) before GMP expansion and banking (Lee and Margolin, 2012).

Immunotherapy holds the potential to induce durable responses, but only a minority of patients currently respond. The etiologies of primary and secondary resistance to immunotherapy are multifaceted, deriving from intrinsic tumour factors and the complex interplay between cancer and its microenvironment (Alcorn et al., 2015). In addressing frontiers in clinical immunotherapy, we describe two categories of approaches to the design of novel drugs and combination therapies: the first involves direct modification of the tumour, at the same time, the second indirectly enhances immunogenicity through alteration of the microenvironment (Alcorn et al., 2015). By systematically addressing the factors that mediate resistance, we can identify mechanistically driven novel approaches to improve immunotherapy outcomes (Alcorn et al., 2015).

Immunotherapy holds the potential to induce durable responses, but only a minority of patients currently respond. The etiologies of primary and secondary resistance to immunotherapy are multifaceted, deriving from intrinsic tumour factors and the complex interplay between cancer and its microenvironment (Igarashi & Sasada, 2020). In addressing frontiers in clinical immunotherapy, we describe two categories of approaches to the design of novel drugs and combination therapies: the first involves direct modification of the tumour, while the second indirectly enhances immunogenicity by altering the microenvironment (Igarashi & Sasada, 2020). By systematically addressing the factors that mediate resistance, we can identify mechanistically-driven novel approaches to improve immunotherapy outcomes (Igarashi & Sasada, 2020).

In addition to surgery, chemotherapy, targeted pathway inhibition and radiation therapy, immunotherapy have emerged as a standard pillar of cancer treatment. Immune checkpoint inhibitors (ICIs) such as those targeting cytotoxic T lymphocyte-associated protein4 (CTLA-4) and programmed cell death protein 1/programmed cell death ligand 1 (PD-1/PD-L1) have been integrated into the standard of care regimens for patients with advanced melanoma (Fong et al., 2021). Merkel cell carcinoma, non-small cell lung cancer, cutaneous squamous cell carcinoma, urothelial cancer, renal cancer, refractory Hodgkin lymphoma, hepatocellular carcinoma, gastric cancer, triple-negative breast cancer, and microsatellite instability (MSI)-high tumours also have been integrated (Fong et al., 2021). Beyond checkpoint inhibitors, cellular therapy in the form of chimeric antigen receptor (CAR) T cells directed at CD19 are now approved in patients with refractory B cell acute lymphoblastic leukemia and large B cell lymphoma. Novel indications and integration of immunotherapy into earlier stages of the disease are being actively investigated (Fong et al., 2021).

Clinical enthusiasm for immunotherapy is high, primarily due to the potential for durable responses, with over 2000 trials ongoing investigating anti-PD-1/anti-PD-L1 targeted drugs alone (Alcorn et al., 2015). However, only a minority of patients treated with immune checkpoint inhibitors (ICIs) respond to these agents. A portion of those patients who do respond will go on to later have progressive, refractory disease (Fong et al., 2021). Primary and acquired resistance necessitates novel agents and combinations. Resistance to immunotherapy is multifaceted. Much attention has been paid to intrinsic tumour factors such as PD-L1 expression, mutational burden, and deficiencies in antigen presentation. Still, the problem of immunotherapy resistance is more complex because tumours exist in a dynamic microenvironment. The tumour microenvironment is a milieu of malignant cells, immune components, blood vessels, extracellular matrix, and signalling molecules that work individually and in combination to influence sensitivity to immunotherapy (Alcorn et al., 2015). Here, we review a variety of strategies to modulate the microenvironment to enhance response to immunotherapy. The approaches fall into two broad categories: direct and indirect modulation of immune-genericity. Natural methods primarily modify the tumour itself, whereas indirect techniques operate predominantly on the microenvironment. These two categories of courses are inextricably linked, with direct modification of the tumour often leading to changes in the microenvironment and vice versa (Fong et al., 2021). We suggest these categorizations as a means to enhance understanding of the primary goal of a particular strategy, and we posit that rational combinations of microenvironment-targeting therapies with ICI or cellular medicine will comprise the next generation of immune-based approaches to cancer treatment (Alcorn et al., 2015). Clinical enthusiasm for immunotherapy is high, primarily due to the potential for durable responses, with over 2000 trials ongoing investigating anti-PD-1/anti-PD-L1 targeted drugs alone (Fong et al., 2021). However, it is only a minority of patients treated with immune checkpoint inhibitors (ICIs) that respond to these agents.

A portion of those patients who do respond will later have progressive, refractory disease. Primary and acquired resistance necessitates novel agents and combinations. Resistance to immunotherapy is multifaceted (Alcorn et al., 2015). Much attention has been paid to intrinsic tumour factors such as PD-L1 expression, mutational burden, and deficiencies in antigen presentation, but the problem of immunotherapy resistance is more complex because tumours exist in a dynamic microenvironment (Alcorn et al., 2015). The tumour microenvironment is a milieu of malignant cells, immune components, blood vessels, extracellular matrix, and signalling molecules that work individually and in combination to influencesensitivity to immunotherapy (Alcorn et al., 2015). Here, we review a variety of strategies to modulate the microenvironment to enhance response to immunotherapy. The approaches fall into two broad categories: direct and indirect modulation of immunogenicity. Natural systems primarily modify the tumour itself, whereas indirect processes operate predominantly on the microenvironment (Alcorn et al., 2015). These two categories of methods are inextricably linked, with direct modification of the tumour often leading to changes in the microenvironment and vice versa (Alcorn et al., 2015). We Suggest these categorizations as a means to enhance understanding of the primary goal of a particular strategy, and we posit that rational combinations of microenvironment-targeting therapies with ICI or cellular medicine will comprise the next generation of immune-based approaches to cancer treatment (Alcorn et al., 2015).

Immunotherapy holds the potential to induce durable responses, but only a minority of patients currently respond. The etiologies of primary and secondary resistance to immunotherapy are multifaceted, deriving from intrinsic tumour factors and the complex interplay between cancer and its microenvironment. In addressing frontiers in clinical immunotherapy, we describe two categories of approaches to the design of novel drugs and combination therapies: the first involves direct modification of the tumour. At the same time, the second indirectly enhances immunogenicity through alteration of the microenvironment. By systematically addressing the factors that mediate resistance, we can identify mechanistically driven novel approaches to improve immunotherapy outcomes (Lee & Margolin, 2012).

Immunotherapy has the ability to produce long-term effects, but only a small percentage of patients respond currently. Primary and secondary immunotherapy resistance have a variety of causes, including tumour intrinsic factors and the dynamic interplay between cancer and its micro-environment (Lee & Margolin, 2012). We define two types of approaches to the design of new drugs and combination therapies in order to resolve clinical immunotherapy frontiers: the first requires direct manipulation of the tumour, while the second indirectly improves immunogenicity by altering the microenvironment. By systematically addressing the variables that mediate resistance, it is possible to overcome it (Lee & Margolin, 2012).

In addition to surgery, chemotherapy, targeted pathway inhibition and radiation therapy, immunotherapy have emerged as a standard pillar of cancer treatment. Immune checkpoint inhibitors (ICIs) such as those targeting cytotoxic T lymphocyte-associated protein 4 (CTLA-4) and programmed cell death protein 1/programmed cell death ligand 1 (PD-1/PD-L1) have been integrated into the standard of care regimens for patients with advanced melanoma, Merkel cell carcinoma, non-small cell lung cancer, cutaneous squamous cell carcinoma, urothelial cancer, renal cancer, refractory Hodgkin lymphoma, hepatocellular carcinoma, gastric cancer, triple-negative breast cancer, and microsatellite instability (MSI)-high tumours (Bordens, 2002). Beyond checkpoint inhibitors, cellular therapy in the form of chimeric antigen receptor (CAR) T cells directed at CD19 are now approved in patients with refractory B cell acute lymphoblastic leukemia and large B cell lymphoma (Bordens, 2002). Novel indications and integration of immunotherapy into earlier stages of the disease are being actively investigated (Bordens, 2002).

Clinical enthusiasm for immunotherapy is high, primarily due to the potential for durable responses, with over 2000 trials ongoing investigating anti-PD-1/anti-PD-L1 targeted drugs alone (Greco, 2020). However, only a minority of patients treated with immune checkpoint inhibitors (ICIs) respond to these agents (Greco, 2020). Furthermore, a portion of those patients who do respond will go on to later have progressive, refractory disease. Thus, primary and acquired resistance necessitates novel agents and combinations (Greco, 2020).

Resistance to immunotherapy is multifaceted. Much attention has been paid to tumour intrinsic factors such as PD-L1 expression, mutational burden, and deficiencies in antigen presentation. Still, the problem of immunotherapy resistance is more complex because tumours exist in a dynamic microenvironment (Greco, 2020). The tumour microenvironment is a milieu of malignant cells, immune components, blood vessels, extracellular matrix, and signalling molecules that work individually and influence sensitivity to immunotherapy (Greco, 2020). Here, we review a variety of strategies to modulate the microenvironment with the goal of enhancing response to immunotherapy. The approaches fall into two broad categories: direct and indirect modulation of immunogenicity. Natural approaches primarily modify the tumour itself, whereas indirect approaches operate predominantly on the microenvironment. These two categories of approaches are inextricably linked, with direct modification of the tumour often leading to changes in the microenvironment and vice versa (Lou, 2018).We suggest these categorizations as a means to enhance understanding of the primary goal of a particular strategy, and we posit that rational combinations of microenvironment-targeting therapies with ICI or cellular therapy will comprise the next generation of immune-based approaches to cancer treatment (Lou, 2018).

To optimize the tumour microenvironment, we must first understand what defines favourable conditions. Immune cells are necessary for an antitumor response, but their presence is insufficient; other mediators play key determining roles. Effector CD8+ T cells [Teff] compete with anti-inflammatory cytokines and cells promoting immune tolerance, including myeloid-derived suppressor cells (MDSC) and regulatory T cells [Tregs]. The Teff/Treg ratio is a prognostic and predictive marker in many tumour types (Lou, 2018).

Solid tumours have been classified as "inflamed" [highly infiltrated with immune cells and proinflammatory cytokines], "immune-deserts" [minimal effector immune cell infiltrate] or the intermediate "immune excluded" [immune cells present in the stroma but not the tumour parenchyma] (Lou, 2018). 10 Inflamed tumours, unsurprisingly, are associated with better clinical outcomes (Lou, 2018). However, CD8+ cell infiltration into the tumour is at best an imperfect marker of immunogenicity, and not all patients with the inflamed phenotype respond to immunotherapy (Lou, 2018). In melanoma patients, baseline CD8+ levels within the tumour are associated with response to PD-1 therapy (Lou, 2018). In contrast, with the anti-CTLA-4 agent ipilimumab, the response is better correlated with post-treatment increases in tumour-infiltrating lymphocytes (TILs) rather than baseline levels (Lou, 2018). This is to say, an inflamed tumour phenotype can promote response, but treatment-induced modulation of a less immunogenic tumour may yield similar results, highlighting opportunities for therapeutic intervention (Lou, 2018).

While defining a tumour's immunogenicity and its microenvironment is challenging, clinical studies have validated several biomarkers. Tumour intrinsic factors, including PD-L1 expression, 11 tumour mutation burden, and mismatch repair deficiency 14 are clinically useful yet imperfect biomarkers because they center around tumour cells (Lou, 2018). We now recognize the pivotal role of the microenvironment, and emerging predictors of responsiveness to anti-PD-1 immunotherapy include associations with T cell receptor (TCR) diversity and/or clonality, host HLA genotype,16 a favourable gut microbiome, and even body mass index, possibly mediated by leptin, among others (Lou, 2018).

UNANSWERED QUESTIONS

There are many unanswered questions when it comes to cancer immunotherapy. The first unanswered question will be if T-cell therapies are used against common solid tumours? T-cell therapy trials have had a lot of success so far, but only in patients with specific blood cancers. According to the American Cancer Society, strong tumours, such as lung, breast, colorectal, pancreatic, and prostate cancers, kill the most people in the United States (Hutch, 2016).

Solid tumours also pose unique problems for immunotherapies that aren't present in liquid tumours. Cancer cells are present in the bloodstream and more open to immune cells, according to several Hutch researchers (Hutch, 2016).

Dr. Ingunn Stromnes, an immunology research associate at Fred Hutch who is developing a T-cell therapy for pancreatic cancer, said, "There are several factors inside the tumour microenvironment that may shut down T cells, and these factors may not be the same for every solid tumour." Interference by other types of immune cells, as well as immunosuppressive signals sent by cancer cells, can block or dampen anti-cancer immune responses in the microscopic environment of a pancreatic tumour, according to Stromnes (Aerts et al., 2014).

Engineering T cells to perceive "shut down" signals as "stay awake" signals is one way to overcome the issue, according to Stromnes. She and her colleagues are currently working on molecules engineered into T cells to do this. She expects preclinical trials to discover a way to boost the anti-cancer response within the year. (Aerts et al., 2014)

Another major problem is determining the best targets for T-cell therapies. Last fall, Stromnes and her Fred Hutch collaborators published the results of a mouse study showing that T cells programmed to destroy pancreatic cancer cells carrying a marker called mesothelin increased survival by more than 75% — a decent number is given that this cancer destroys the majority of its human victims with (Hutch, 2016).

"We're going to bring T cells into the clinic as soon as possible," Stromnes said, "because we think we have something that will work."

Researchers can now sequence the genomes of individual tumours rapidly and affordably thanks to new technology, which was previously impossible. Multiple groups in the Hutch and worldwide are looking for T-cell targets in various tumour forms, thanks to effective genomic sequencing (Hutch, 2016).

Is it possible to get more patients to benefit from targeted immune-boosting drugs? Immune checkpoint inhibitors, which block signals that suppress T cells' cancer-killing activity, are another form of immunotherapy becoming more common. These medications have shown to be highly successful in some patients. Immune checkpoint inhibitors, which block signals that suppress T cells' cancer-killing activity, are another form of immunotherapy becoming more common. These medications have shown to be highly successful in some patients.

These medications, however, are only effective in a small percentage of patients. How do more people benefit from them?

Dr. Mary "Nora" Disis, a solid tumour immunotherapist at the University of Washington and Fred Hutch explained that most cancers do not cause much of an immune response, to begin with (Xu et al., 2020).

And new research indicates that patients who already have anti-cancer immune responses respond better to these medications. In this situation, Disis believes that finding ways to activate an immune response within a tumour, which can then be strengthened with a checkpoint inhibitor, would be the answer. She believes that some currently available drugs, such as immune-stimulating chemotherapies, may play this role (Hutch, 2016).

"We now need to look at several factors that have been shown to improve immunity and reflect on how we can incorporate immunotherapy into the standard of care now," Disis said. According to Dr. Lee Cranmer, director of Hutch's Bob and Eileen Gilman Family Sarcoma Research Program, the opposite issue is also essential.

"We don't want to give patients stuff with possible toxicities without being able to concentrate them better," Cranmer said, who has worked on checkpoint inhibitor clinical trials. "One of our goals (in the field) is to take what we already have and say, 'ok, how do we target [this treatment] on those who are most likely to gain,' rather than saying, 'ok, let's just throw something at you and see if it works.'" What are the risks associated with cancer immunotherapy? (Hutch, 2016).

Cancer immunotherapy, like any other drug or medical treatment, may cause side effects. The types and severity of side effects you encounter are determined by various factors, including your physical health, the type of cancer being treated, the drug used, and how it is administered, fever, chills, exhaustion, nausea, diarrhea, body aches, and fatigue are typical flu-like symptoms associated with cancer immunotherapy (Xu et al., 2020).

Many immunotherapy drugs may cause a rash and itchiness on your skin. This may occur during your treatment and may persist after you have completed it. If you notice any of these changes on your skin, talk to your doctor, they may recommend creams or medications to help alleviate the itching. (Hutch, 2016).

Before beginning treatment, talk to your doctor about the potential side effects. Notify your doctor right away if you encounter any side effects during your procedure. He or she will be able to find ways to help you mitigate or control your side effects so that you can get through your care with as little discomfort as possible (Hutch, 2016).

Another unanswered question about immunotherapy is the use in patients with metastatic bladder cancer? Over the past decade, chemotherapy has been the first-line treatment for metastatic bladder cancer, either cisplatin-based chemotherapy in patients who are cisplatin eligible or carboplatin-based chemotherapy in patients who are not cisplatin eligible. Chemotherapy has a response rate of 30 to 50 percent in patients with metastatic bladder cancer, as we all know. A small percentage of patients, especially those receiving cisplatin-based chemotherapy, will have long-lasting responses, but most patients will improve.

In the past, there were no global standard therapies for patients with bladder cancer who progressed after receiving first-line chemotherapy. However, thanks to the advancement of immune checkpoint inhibitors, five PD-1 and PD-L1 inhibitors are now approved for the second-line treatment of metastatic bladder cancer that has progressed despite first-line chemotherapy (Hutch, 2016).

As a result, a big issue has arisen: Should these medications be moved earlier in the treatment process? Should we combine them with chemotherapy because they seem to be non-cross resistant to chemotherapy and have non-overlapping toxicity profiles? It has essentially resulted in two main questions being answered in two massive, international randomized trials.

One issue is whether patients with metastatic bladder cancer can receive immune checkpoint blockade in addition to chemotherapy or immune checkpoint blockade alone.

Patients in the IMvigor study are randomly assigned to either standard of care chemotherapy or gemcitabine and cisplatin, regardless of whether they are cisplatin-ineligible or not. It is choosing between conventional chemotherapy, chemotherapy with a PD-L1 inhibitor, and single-agent chemotherapy (Hutch, 2016). So, it'll be three-arm randomization to see whether immunotherapy, chemotherapy or a combination of the two should be provided to this patient population. The second main question that emerges, based on data from platinum-resistant patients and, of course, data from other solid tumours, is: Should we offer combination immunotherapy that includes CTLA-4 blockade and PD-1 or PD-L1 blockade? (Igarashi & Sasada, 2020).

Combination immunotherapy can increase the response rate compared to single-agent chemotherapy in other solid tumours such as melanoma, kidney cancer, and, more recently, lung cancer. These reactions are usually long-lasting. Thus, in the platinum-resistant setting in bladder cancer, a combination of CTLA-4 blockade and PD-1 blockade has been studied, with response rates that appear to be slightly higher than PD-1 blockade alone, raising the question of whether we should be providing doublet immune checkpoint blockade to patients with metastatic bladder cancer as a first-line treatment. As a result, the CheckMate-901 analysis is putting this theory to the test. Since the randomization is done differently depending on whether patients are cisplatin eligible or disqualified, it's a little more complicated in this study. The study's primary endpoint is focused on the cisplatin-ineligible population, and those patients are randomized to either standard of care chemotherapy or a combination of [Yervoy (ipilimumab)] and [Opdivo (nivolumab)]. (Valenti et al., 2021)

There is three-arm randomization for cisplatin-ineligible patients, with patients being assigned to (Yervoy) plus (Opdivo) versus standard of care chemotherapy plus (Opdivo) (Opdivo). So, once again, a study has the potential to alter the standard of care for first-line metastatic bladder cancer. What is the condition of the trials right now? Both tests are currently recruiting participants. The accrual will take some time to complete, and patients will be monitored before the primary endpoint is reached. Can you see chemotherapy being phased out of the treatment of bladder cancer in the future? I see a lot in which chemotherapy plays a smaller role in bladder cancer care, but I don't think it'll go away anytime soon. If the clinical trials turn out to be what we hope they will be, I believe the combination of chemotherapy and immune checkpoint blockade will help at least some patients. At least for certain patients, this would be normal treatment. I think it's a fascinating topic whether chemotherapy alone will play a part in the treatment of bladder cancer in the future. I believe it is true that it would not. What would you think the current takeaway from these studies is? The lesson from the first-line trials in metastatic bladder cancer is that the questions being posed are very realistic, straightforward questions that can only be answered in the form of a large randomized clinical trial.

Is single-agent immunotherapy, doublet immunotherapy, chemotherapy combinations, or chemotherapy alone the potential (of bladder cancer treatment)? We may make all the assumptions we want, but the only way to know for sure is to conduct prospective clinical trials (Hutch, 2016).

Which immunotherapy regimen can lung cancer patients undergo as a first-line treatment?

Oncologists had evidence that Keytruda helped some patients with metastatic NSCLC live longer when they presented at ASCO. However, concerns remained about which patients would benefit more from receiving Keytruda alone and those who would benefit most from receiving Keytruda combined with chemotherapy. Two-Phase three trials of Keytruda presented at this year's conference help to paint a clearer picture, highlighting the mainstay role Keytruda appears to play in initial disease care (Hutch, 2016).

Keytruda is currently the only immunotherapy approved for the treatment of NSCLC as a first-line treatment. The PD-1 inhibitor is approved as a monotherapy for patients with PD-L1 protein expression greater than 50% and as a combination therapy for all patients with nonsquamous NSCLC (Hutch, 2016).

In patients with the harder-to-treat squamous type of NSCLC, combining Keytruda with a separate chemo regimen also improved survival, regardless of PD-L1 expression, according to new evidence. This indicated that Keytruda plus chemotherapy is a better choice than chemotherapy alone for all NSCLC patients without a driver mutation like EGFR or ALK. A second study comparing Keytruda to chemotherapy in NSCLC patients with more than 1% PD-L1 expression drew a lot of interest at the meeting. In the narrowly selected patient population, the trial showed that Keytruda monotherapy decreased the risk of dying compared to chemo. However, responses among patients with elevated PD-L1 levels were responsible for a large portion of the survival gain. "The higher PD-L1 subgroup is clearly driving this advantage," said Gandhi of NYU. "The advantage is not as apparent for those with 1% to 49%, where a much greater number of patients do not benefit from immunotherapy," says the researcher (Xu et al., 2020).

However, Keytruda was found to be much less toxic than chemotherapy, meaning that it could be useful for patients who aren't good candidates for chemotherapy. In an interview, Gilberto Lopes, the lead researcher on the second Keytruda trial, said that medical consensus will likely coalesce around giving immunotherapy with chemo to patients who express PD-L1 between 1% and 49% while opting for Keytruda alone in PD-L1 high people. However, ongoing studies of checkpoint inhibitors by Merck's competitors Roche and Bristol-Myers could complicate the approach. (Valenti et al., 2021)

Bristol-Myers Squibb is working on a combination of two immunotherapies, Opdivo and Yervoy, that could provide a chemo-free choice for patients who express a biomarker called tumour mutation burden. The role of immunotherapy in first-line lung cancer treatment, however, is clear. In remarks delivered during a plenary session, Gandhi said, "Chemotherapy alone is no longer a first-line standard of treatment in non-small cell lung cancer."

Is it possible that companies have rushed into large-scale trials of immunotherapy combinations?

The industry's recent investment in cancer research has focused on combining immunotherapies with other treatments. There are currently over 1,100 ongoing combination studies using the five licenced checkpoint inhibitors (Hutch, 2016).

Aside from immunotherapy and chemo combinations, much of this study has yielded few clear-cut successes. For example, a closely followed Phase 3 trial in melanoma of Incyte's IDO inhibitor epacadostat and Keytruda failed earlier this year, demonstrating that Incyte's drug provided little additional value. It was a devastating blow to one of the industry's most advanced combinations, raising concerns about whether the two drugmakers acted too fast. Investors are now concerned that another high-profile merger might take the same route. On Monday, Nektar Therapeutics' market capitalization dropped $6 billion as investors digested a muddled report on the biotech's experimental drug NKTR-214 and Opdivo combination. The partners approved three late-stage trials of the two drugs in melanoma, kidney, and bladder cancers, based on positive results from a small number of patients (Hutch, 2016).

The decision raised questions about whether the companies had enough evidence to proceed to Phase 3, particularly when the second group of patients didn't seem to have the same high level of response. It's a dilemma that the entire field is grappling with, as businesses weigh the benefits of waiting for more (or any) randomized data against moving forward with pairings that have a good biologic justification (Hutch, 2016).

"Have you accumulated enough translational data?" Are we following in the footsteps of IDO, investing millions of dollars on a large number of patients from the beginning to the end? Others, on the other hand, say that it's worth investing in when there's ample proof of good potential (Hutch, 2016).

In an interview, Kim Blackwell, head of early-phase oncology growth at Eli Lilly, said, "It's really easy to say any asset needs a randomized Phase 2 before moving into Phase 3." "However, if you have good science and a safe agent in the early stages, going straight to a large clinical trial can get you there faster. Better treatments are needed for our patients." (Igarashi & Sasada, 2020).

Immunotherapy has a number of advantages over traditional treatments including chemotherapy and radiation, including short- and long-term side effects. The desire to continue care for an extended period of time while maintaining a high standard of living is a huge cost (Hutch, 2016).

Standard cancer treatments can cure certain cancers, but they may also have long-term side effects including peripheral neuropathy, heart problems, surgical complications, lung damage, hormone dysfunction, and memory and cognitive issues. Normal therapies can eventually cause the immune system to be compromised or overpowered (Valenti et al., 2021).

FUTURE PERSPECTIVES OF CANCER IMMUNOTHERAPY

As supported by the previous chapters, cancer immunotherapy is a complicated, dynamic, and vital field of research. Each research specialty faces unique challenges with the application of immunotherapy, but there are promising leads to effective treatment. The future of cancer immunotherapy depends on continued efforts to learn more about the disease and the drive to innovate new solutions. There are several future perspectives on exploring cancer immunotherapy, from immune system imaging to holistic approaches to human health.

In the past, cancer treatment in Canada has been managed through one primary oncologist to treat the disease through radiation, chemotherapy, and surgery (Tagliaferri et al., 2020). However, treatment in Canada has turned to a more holistic approach to give the patient every advantage to recover from this disease. Holistic cancer treatment typically involves not only a medical oncologist but also a healthcare team including a family doctor, occupational therapist, nurse and oncology-specific nurse, palliative care clinic, pathologist, pharmacist, physiotherapist, radiation oncologist as well as radiation therapist, speech-language pathologist, psychiatrist, dietitian, and social worker or counsellor (Forbes et al., 2019). Each patient may have a different healthcare team that can help increase the immunotherapy efficacy and ease the patient's experience through collaboration and communication. This basis of personalized healthcare impacts every aspect of treatment and the potential capabilities of the immunotherapy treatment itself.

Monotherapy is the use of a single-agent antibody, cell type, or sequence to induce the patient's immune system to halt the proliferation of cancer cells. This is the foundation of immunotherapy treatment and therefore, innovation will continue through this strategy of treatment. There are two main directions of research that will yield new treatments. The first is to discover new targets within the cancer cells for immune recognition as 'non-self' (Ralli et al., 2020). These new targets are essential for targeting specific types of cancer cells and more effectively halting their proliferation. For example, melanoma is a variable form of cancer that can develop and spread in many different ways (Valenti et al., 2021). Researchers are looking for new genes such as LAG3, TIM3, OX-40, CD137, IDO, and GITR for the immune system to recognize and destroy (Ralli et al., 2020). Different targets allow more opportunities to correctly identify the cancer cells and prevent adverse effects in healthy cells. Another aspect of monotherapy's future directions is to search for new methods to induce the immune system to respond to cancer. For example, nivolumab is a human monoclonal antibody that targets the programmed cell death ligand 1 (PD-1), a cell division checkpoint in cancer cells (Reck et al., 2018). It is a promising start as a third-line treatment, but international studies have reported different efficacy levels from 4.7% to 20.6% overall response rates (Reck et al., 2018). This is one example of hundreds of immunotherapy treatments that require more clinical trials and development to be considered safe and effective. Monotherapy is a good starting point for the continued development of immunotherapy treatment. However, researchers are finding promising leads in combining different treatments for a more holistic approach.

Combination therapy is the use of multiple strategies to treat and prevent the spread of cancer. Immunotherapy treatments can be used in concert with each other or with other treatment methods. Using multiple immunotherapy drugs induces the immune system to target various cancer cell-division checkpoints at once, increasing the ability of the immune system to recognize and stop cancer cells (Huang et al., 2021). For example, nivolumab as monotherapy has presently demonstrated minimal impact. However, in combination with ipilimumab, another checkpoint targeting immunotherapy, there has been more success in the immune response. One study on small cell lung cancer (SCLC) observed an overall response rate of 10% with nivolumab alone and 33% combined with ipilimumab immune checkpoint inhibitor (ICI) therapy (Antonia et al., 2016). This is an improved response compared to nivolumab on its own, demonstrating that the immune system can be induced to target multiple checkpoints with multiple ICIs at the same time. While it is not a complete solution, the results of this study support the future potential for ICI combined immunotherapy.

Another branch of combined immunotherapy is chemoradiotherapy (chemotherapy and radiotherapy) in concert with the immunotherapy agents. Combining immunotherapy with chemoradiotherapy increases tumour antigens' release, which allows the immunotherapy to work more rapidly and effectively (Huang et al., 2021). In SCLC, response to current chemotherapy (platinum etoposide doublet) has been positive with about 70% response; relapse occurs in approximately 80% of limited-stage lung cancer patients and all extensive stage lung cancer patients (Puglisi et al., 2010). There has been very little success with second-line treatment (single-agent topotecan) and no applicable third line of therapy past the clinical trial stage (Huang et al., 2021). I have made progress in treating tumours by targeting checkpoints in cell division and halting rapid cellular division. The challenge with SCLC is that the ICIs have had low success targeting the PD-L1 checkpoint due to low expression and T-cell interference (Hamilton and Rath, 2019). Combining ICI immunotherapy with chemoradiotherapy and other ICIs has demonstrated promise in overcoming these challenges (Sen et al., 2019). For example, the use of the chemotherapy drug cisplatin on SCLC has been proven to activate NK cells, which are immune effectors (Gasser et al., 2005). Cisplatin can also disrupt transcription and expression of programmed cell death receptor-ligand 2 on dendritic cells as well as tumour cells, which decreases immunosuppression by tumour cells (Lesterhuis et al., 2011). Both functions of this chemotherapy treatment assist the function of immunotherapy agents in halting the proliferation of cancer cells. Similarly, radiotherapy treatments have been proven to boost the effect of immunotherapy. In melanoma combined treatments, specialists have observed that the regression of tumour lesions after radiation treatment is increased when combined with immunotherapy (Pfannenstiel et al., 2019). Further to this, radiation treatments cause the immune response to intensifying due to the exposure of identifying molecules and an increase in inflammatory cell recruitment to the irradiated area (Weichselbaum et al., 2017). While combined chemoradiotherapy with immunotherapy may not produce results in all forms of cancer, it is an avenue for more efficient and effective immunotherapy treatment going forward (Huang et al., 2021). Combined immunotherapy is an important future perspective in cancer research, and due to the differences in genetic makeup, the precise treatment regimen is becoming more personalized.

Personal oncogenomics is the cutting edge of cancer research today. Because cancer cells begin in the patient's own cells, understanding the patient's genetic makeup can inform researchers on the best treatment strategy. This also plays into the function of immunotherapy using the patient's own immune system. For example, patients with paraneoplastic syndromes such as Lambert-Eaton syndrome have demonstrated more sensitivity to ICI immunotherapy than patients without genetic disorders (Ivanovski and Miralles, 2019). Further to this, patients with neurological paraneoplastic syndromes have also demonstrated a more robust lymphocyte response to tumours, resulting in a better answer to treatment (Iams et al., 2019). These genetic syndromes and their respective positive response to immunotherapy illustrate how vital genetic information is to the future development of immunotherapy treatments. Next-generation sequencing (NGS) can provide insight into what mutations in the DNA have caused the uncontrolled proliferation of the cells, which can help identify which targets might be most effective for immunotherapy (Gupta et al., 2016). A model to predict immunotherapy treatment response has been developed, called an immunotherapy score (ITS) (Jiang et al., 2020). The ITS examines the exome (exons of the genome expressed) for specific biomarkers connected to suitable responses to immunotherapy treatments such as NF-kB negative regulators (Amato et al., 2020). With the continued development of these genetic suitability markers, immunotherapy can become more safe and suitable for cancer treatment.

Beyond genomics studying DNA, there are also multi-omic analyses that can inform researchers of new pharmacological targets and assist in predicting the outcome of different immunotherapy treatments. Multi-omics includes proteomics, metabolomics, radionics, transcriptomics, and genomics (Valenti et al., 2021). Transcriptomics is the study of the transcriptome, which includes mRNA (Valenti et al., 2021). The current use of transcriptomics is the Immuno-Predictive Score (IMPRES). This score uses 15 transcriptomic relationships between immune checkpoint genes to predict response to ICIs (Auslander et al., 2018). While IMPRES is a promising start to predict how a patient will react to ICI, some forms of cancer, such as the highly variable melanoma, remain challenging to predict despite decoding mRNA (Valenti et al., 2021). Continued research into more unpredictable forms of cancer and new transcriptomic relationships (Valenti et al., 2021). Proteomics is the study of proteins that can provide important information about tumour cells and healthy cells. Studies have demonstrated differences in the proteins of the patients who responded to immunotherapy and those who did not, particularly in lipid and ketone metabolism as well as plasmatic PD-1 (Harel et al., 2019; Babačić et al., 2020). Proteomics may also provide future insight into biomarkers of toxicity and irAEs, a crucial aspect of immunotherapy that still requires much research. Metabolomics is another area of study that can help identify cellular health by observing changes in low molecular weight products of cells (Valenti et al., 2021). Cancer cells can produce molecules that are not produced in healthy cells due to the altered state of growth. LDH is a melanoma-specific biomarker involved in converting pyruvate to lactate. Increased cell necrosis causes LDH to enter the bloodstream at elevated levels, determining prognosis factors and potential drug responses. Studies have begun to explore the relationship between various metabolite levels in the bloodstream and immunotherapy response. Metabolomics is an 'omic' area with a high potential for future research (Valenti et al., 2021). Radiomics is a medical approach to deciphering tumour features from radiological biomedical images, which are instrumental in defining the quantitative progress of the disease (Valenti et al., 2021). Radiomics bridges the gap between medicine and machine learning, making it a very exciting prospect as medical technology improves in the future.

Radiomics plays a vital role in imaging the severity and progression of cancer tumours. These images are created through Computed Tomography (CT), Magnetic Resonance Imaging (MRI), or Positron Emission Tomography (PET) scans (Aerts et al., 2014). These images are useful in determining the success or failure of immunology treatments. However, it can be challenging to determine what the results actually indicate about the patient's response to the treatment strategy. Immunotherapy treatments can display a pseudoprogression wherein there is an increase of tumour growth before the treatment takes effect (Nishino et al., 2018). It is imperative to monitor this pseudoprogression as it can have adverse effects on patient health. Radiologists play an essential role in communicating the implications of increased tumour growth throughout an immunotherapy treatment. Deciphering the meaning of these tumour response dynamics can be complicated considering it may be weeks to months between a positive immune response and a reduction in tumour size and number. As well, a positive immune response to treatment may indicate that the agent is effective in halting the spread of cancer cells but may not indicate patient survival.

Beyond understanding pseudoprogression in tumour response dynamics, it is also important to be cognizant of potential immune-related adverse events (irAEs) in radiological imaging (Nishino et al., 2018). These irAEs involve toxicity responses in the patient's immune system, which occur when the patient's immune system is misdirected in immunotherapy and begins targeting healthy cells (Baxi et al., 2018). For example, hypophysitis is an irAE associated with the agent ipilimumab, which causes endocrine system dysfunction (Barra-Sousa et al., 2018). In the case of hypophysitis, MRI image resolution becomes instrumental in identifying the detrimental pituitary enlargement associated with ipilimumab (Nishino et al., 2018). Prognosis of the development of irAEs can become challenging when using combination immunotherapy because one or both of the agents may be responsible for causing the irAEs. As the number of immunotherapy agents increases, radiologists need to recognize the signs of irAEs in each case and work collaboratively with the treatment team to manage the irAEs. Looking to the future, radiological imaging continues to face challenges with high levels of background signals making the desired region challenging to delineate and non-specific uptake resulting in long time intervals between injection of radioactive particles and visualization on an MRI (Mayer et al., 2017). These obstacles may be overcome with continued collaboration and research, but not without a robust funding system.

Even in countries like Canada, which has a government-funded healthcare system, experimental treatments rely greatly on philanthropy. Much of the experimental treatments, such as new immunotherapy targets or combinations, require charitable donations to create everything from the physical lab space to the antigen sourcing (Nelson, 2017). Checkpoint blockade immunotherapy costs approximately $100k/treatment cycle to produce and utilize (Nelson, 2017). The donation model presents a problem because it can be challenging to predict sufficient funds from year to year, and donors may dictate which area of research or care their funds go to support. For example, the Conconi Family Immunotherapy Lab in British Columbia produces essential custom immunotherapy treatments using Chimeric Antigen Receptor -T cells (Nelson, 2017). This lab runs primarily with donated funds to produce this life-saving treatment. Another arena for immunotherapy funding has been BioCanRx, a hub for Canadian immunotherapy networking. BioCanRx is funded mainly by the Networks of Centres of Excellence Program through the federal government as well as corporate partners (Nelson, 2017). BioCanRx is funding research to develop and refine new monotherapy targets, new combination approaches, more robust policy frameworks to apply the immunotherapeutics, and better early health technology assessments (Birdie et al., 2021; Murdoch, 2020; Salim et al., 2020). These projects represent many of the critical leads discussed in immunotherapy research. Personalized cancer treatment and immunotherapy research is a well-funded cancer research area due to its application across many types of cancer. However, experimental medical research must continue to be financially supported as long as there are promising future perspectives to investigate.

There are many exciting prospects in the works for improving immunotherapy efficacy and safety. Looking to the future, treatment plans are becoming more personalized and collaborative. The improvements in monotherapy can lead to improvements in combined immunotherapy and chemoradiotherapy approaches. Detailed multi-omics are opening the door to earlier prognosis and scalability of immunotherapy success, as well as better toxicity predictions. The harmonious development of radiomics is already improving the ability of a medical treatment team to react to changes in immunotherapy responses. The prevention of irAEs will continue to improve as further medical and technological advancements are made in both radiomics and immunotherapy treatments themselves. Finally, the continued financial support, be through private, corporate, or government funding, is instrumental in securing the future advancements of immunotherapy treatments. The nature of cancer is to mutate and change, constantly presenting new challenges to immunotherapy treatment plans. If we want to leave the threat of cancer in the past, we need to continue innovating and collaborating to build a better future.

Sabika Sami

CONCLUSION

Cancer immunotherapy is a complicated and promising addition to getting rid of cancerous cells in the human body. Before, Cancer was prevented with various techniques that garnered an assault on human tissues and overall health (Schuster, 2006). A combination of chemotherapy, radiation or surgery can commonly treat cancer through its localized sites. However, it is not effective as cancerous cells can travel and affect the whole body (Schuster, 2006). So it is in critical conditions where another more effective eradication technique comes into play, immunotherapy. Discovered by William B. Coley, immunotherapy strengthens the body's immune system with cells that already prevent it within the human body; that is to say, the method of immunotherapeutic treatment is conducted only by how well the immune system can conduct it (Schuster, 2006). Immunotherapy is produced based on the immune system cells, such as the T cells, which block or activate regulatory receptions using antibodies and prevent further disease progression (Schuster, 2006). The main cancer immunotherapy strategies try to eradicate tumour-related antibodies by combined cytotoxic and humoral cell effector mechanisms by the host immune system (Schuster, 2006). With new technology and science, the battle of cancer is slowly diminishing out, but one must also remember the social impact cancer has on society. Regardless of race, gender, or class, cancer is a known killer in our society. However, studies suggest that differences in societal status are responsible for cancer occurrence, mainly among the lower portion of the population than the higher, more wealthy populations (Baquet, 1991). As mentioned in chapter 1, understanding the social determinants of health regarding cancer is imperative for the future prevention of the disease. Taking initiative to find one of the manageable root causes for illness and changing it is similar to immunotherapy itself. When understanding where and why an uprising of disease is coming from and taking it upon oneself to change and tackle the root of the problem, we can genuinely solve cancer, not just cure it.

WORKS CITED

Abbott, M., & Ustoyev, Y. (2019). Cancer and the Immune System: The History and Background of Immunotherapy. Seminars In Oncology Nursing, 35(5), 150923 DOI: 10.1016/j.soncn.2019.08.002

Acevedo, J.A.M., Dholaria, B., Soyano, A.E., Knutson, K.L., Chumsri, S., & Lou, Y. (2018). Next-generation of immune checkpoint therapy in cancer: new developments and challenges. Journal of Hematology and Oncology, 11(39). DOI: 10.1186/s13045-018-0582-8

Aerts, H. J. W. L., Velazquez, E. R., Leijenaar, R. T. H., Parmar, C., Grossmann, P., Carvalho, S., Bussink, J., Monshouwer, R., Haibe-Kains, B., Rietveld, D., Hoebers, F., & Lambin, P. (2014). Erratum: Corrigendum: Decoding tumour phenotype by noninvasive imaging using a quantitative radiomics approach. Nature Communications, 5(1). DOI:10.1038/ncomms5644

Alcorn, J., Burton, R., & Topping, A. (2015). BCG treatment for bladder cancer, from past to present use. International Journal of Urological Nursing, 9(3), 177-186. DOI: 10.1111/ijun.12064

Allison, J. P., & Krummel, M. F. (1995). The Yin and Yang of T cell costimulation. Science, 270(5238), 932-932. DOI: 10.1126/science.270.5238.932

Amato, C. M., Hintzsche, J. D., Wells, K., Applegate, A., Gorden, N. T., Vorwald, V. M., Tobin, R.P., Nassar, K., Shellman, Y.G., Kim, J., and Medina, T.M. (2020). Pre-Treatment Mutational and Transcriptomic Landscape of Responding Metastatic Melanoma Patients to Anti-PD1 Immunotherapy. Cancers, 12(7), 1943. DOI: 10.3390/cancers12071943

Antonia, S. J., López-Martin, J. A., Bendell, J., Ott, P. A., Taylor, M., Eder, J. P., Jäger, D., Pietanza, M.C., Le, D.T., de Braud, F., Morse, M.A. & Calvo, E. (2016). Nivolumab alone and nivolumab plus ipilimumab in recurrent small-cell lung cancer (CheckMate 032): a multicentre, open-label, phase 1/2 trial. The Lancet Oncology, 17(7), 883–895. DOI:10.1016/s1470-2045(16)30098-5

Auslander, N., Zhang, G., Lee, J. S., Frederick, D. T., Miao, B., Moll, T., Tian, T., Wei, Z., Madan, S., Sullivan, R.J., Boland, G., & Ruppin, E. (2018). Robust prediction of response to immune checkpoint blockade therapy in metastatic melanoma. Nature

Medicine, 24(10), 1545–1549.
DOI: 10.1038/s41591-018-0157-9

Babačić, H., Lehtiö, J., Pico de Coaña, Y., Pernemalm, M., & Eriksson, H. (2020). In-depth plasma proteomics reveals an increase in circulating PD-1 during anti-PD-1 immunotherapy in patients with metastatic cutaneous melanoma. Journal for ImmunoTherapy of Cancer, 8(1). DOI: 10.1136/jitc-2019-000204

Bagherifar, R., Kiaie, S. H., Hatami, Z., Ahmadi, A., Sadeghnejad, A., Baradaran, B.,Javadzadeh, Y. (2021). Nanoparticle-mediated synergistic chemoimmunotherapy for tailoring cancer therapy: recent advances and perspectives. Journal of Nanobiotechnology, 19(1). DOI: 10.1186/s12951-021-00861-0

Baldwin, R. (1955). Immunity to Methylcholanthrene-Induced Tumours in Inbred Rats Following Atrophy and Regression of the Implanted Tumours. British Journal Of Cancer, 9(4), 652-657.
DOI: 10.1038/bjc.1955.70

Baquet, C. R., Horm, J. W., Gibbs, T., & Greenwald, P. (1991). Socioeconomic Factors and Cancer Incidence Among Blacks and Whites. JNCI Journal of the National Cancer Institute, 83(8), 551–557.
DOI: 10.1093/jnci/83.8.551

Barroso-Sousa, R., Barry, W. T., Garrido-Castro, A. C., Hodi, F. S., Min, L., Krop, I. E., & Tolaney, S. M. (2018). Incidence of Endocrine Dysfunction Following the Use of Different Immune Checkpoint Inhibitor Regimens. JAMA Oncology, 4(2), 173.
DOI: 10.1001/jamaoncol.2017.3064

Baxi, S., Yang, A., Gennarelli, R. L., Khan, N., Wang, Z., Boyce, L., & Korenstein, D. (2018). Immune-related adverse events for anti-PD-1 and anti-PD-L1 drugs: systematic review and meta-analysis. BMJ.
DOI: 10.1136/bmj.k793

Bendle, G. M., Linnemann, C., Hooijkaas, A. I., Bies, L., de Witte, M. A., Jorritsma, A., M Kaiser, A. D., Pouw, N., Debets, R., Kieback, E., Uckert, W., Song, J.-Y., A G Haanen, J. B., & M Schumacher, T. N. (2010). Lethal graft-versus-host disease in mouse models of T cell receptor gene therapy. Nature Medicine.
DOI: 10.1038/nm.2128

Benz, T. A. (2019). Toxic Cities: Neoliberalism and Environmental Racism in Flint and Detroit Michigan. Critical Sociology, 45(1), 49–62.
DOI: 10.1177/0896920517708339

Birdi, H. K., Jirovec, A., Cortés-Kaplan, S., Werier, J., Nessim, C., Diallo, J. S., & Ardolino, M. (2021). Immunotherapy for sarcomas: new frontiers and unveiled opportunities. Journal for Immunotherapy of Cancer, 9(2).
DOI: 10.1136/jitc-2020-001580

Botticelli , A., Visconti, I. C., Angeletti, D., Fiore , M., Marchetti , P., Lambiase , A., Lambiase, A., de Vincentiis, M., & Greco, A. (2020). Immunotherapy in the Treatment of Metastatic Melanoma: Current Knowledge and Future Directions.
DOI: 10.1155/2020/9235638

Brassard, D. L., Grace, M. J., & Bordens, R. W. (2002). Interferon-α as an immunothera-peutic protein. Journal of leukocyte biology, 71(4), 565-581.
DOI: 10.1189/jlb.71.4.565

Bullock, T. N. J. (2021). Fundamentals of cancer immunology and their application to cancer vaccines. Clinical and Translational Science, 14(1), 120-131.
DOI: 10.1111/cts.12856

Burnet, M., & Fenner, F. (1949). The Production of Antibodies. London: Macmillan.

Burnet, M. (1957). Cancer--A Biological Approach: III. Viruses Associated with Neoplas-tic Conditions. IV. Practical Applications. BMJ, 1(5023), 841-847.
DOI: 10.1136/bmj.1.5023.841

Burnet, F. M. (1967). Immunological aspects of malignant disease. The Lancet, 289(7501), 1171-1174.
DOI: 10.1016/S0140-6736(67)92837-1

Calne, R. Y., Thiru, S., McMaster, P., Craddock, G. N., White, D. J. G., Evans, D. B., ... & Rolles, K. (1978). Cyclosporin A in patients receiving renal allografts from cadaver donors. The Lancet, 312(8104), 1323-1327.
DOI: 10.1016/S0140-6736(78)91970-0

Campbell, C., Greenberg, R., Mankikar, D., & Ross, R. (2016). A Case Study of Environ-mental Injustice: The Failure in Flint. International Journal of Environmental Research and Public Health, 13(10), 951. MDPI AG.
DOI: 10.3390/ijerph13100951

Cancer Immunotherapy Timeline of Progress. (2021). Retrieved 7 May 2021, from https://www.cancerresearch.org/immunotherapy/timeline-of-progress

Chakraborty, S., & Rahman, T. (2012). The difficulties in cancer treatment. Ecancer-medicalscience, 6, ed16.
DOI: 10.3332/ecancer.2012.ed16

Chen, E. H., Shofer, F. S., Dean, A. J., Hollander, J. E., Baxt, W. G., Robey, J. L., Sease, K. L., & Mills, A. M. (2008). Gender disparity in analgesic treat-ment of emergency department patients with acute abdominal pain. Academic emergency medicine: official journal of the Society for Academic Emergency Medicine, 15(5), 414–418.
DOI: 10.1111/j.1553-2712.2008.00100.x

Coley, W. B. (1893). The Treatment of Malignant tumours by Repeated Inoculations of Erysipelas. The American Journal of the Medical Sciences, 105(5), 487–510.
DOI: 10.1097/00000441-189305000-00001

Coulie, P. G., van den Eynde, B. J., van der Bruggen, P., & Boon, T. (2014). Tumour antigens recognized by T lymphocytes: At the core of cancer immunotherapy. In Nature Reviews Cancer (Vol. 14, Issue 2, pp. 135–146). Nature Publishing Group.
DOI: 10.1038/nrc3670

Creelan, B.C. Update on immune checkpoint inhibitors in lung cancer. (2014). Cancer Control, 21(1), 80-9.
DOI: 10.1177/107327481402100112.

Dalakas M. C. (2018). Neurological complications of immune checkpoint inhibitors: what happens when you 'take the brakes off the immune system. Therapeutic advances in neurological disorders, 11, 1756286418799864.
DOI: 10.1177/1756286418799864

Delves, P., & Roitt, I. (2000). The Immune System. New England Journal Of Medicine, 343(1), 37-49.
DOI: 10.1056/nejm200007063430107

Dobosz, P., & Dzieciątkowski, T. (2019). The Intriguing History of Cancer Immunotherapy. Frontiers In Immunology, 10.
DOI: 10.3389/fimmu.2019.02965

Donia, M., Junker, N., Ellebaek, E., Andersen, M. H., Straten, P. T., & Svane, I. M. (2012). Characterization and comparison of "standard" and "young" tumour-infiltrating lymphocytes for adoptive cell therapy at a danish translational research institution. Scandinavian Journal of Immunology, 75(2), 157–167.
DOI: 10.1111/j.1365-3083.2011.02640.x

Dudley, M. E., Wunderlich, J. R., Robbins, P. F., Yang, J. C., Hwu, P., Schwartzentruber, D. J., Topalian, S. L., Sherry, R., Restifo, N. P., Hubicki, A. M., Robinson, M. R., Raffeld, M., Duray, P., Seipp, C. A., Rogers-Freezer, L., Morton, K. E., Mavroukakis, S. A., White, D. E., & Rosenberg, S. A. (2002). Cancer regression and autoimmunity in patients after clonal repopulation with antitumour lymphocytes. Science, 298(5594), 850–854.
DOI: 10.1126/science.1076514

Ehrlich P. (1897). Die Wertbesmessung des Diphterieilserums und deren theoretische Grundlagen [The measurement of diphtheria serum and its theoretical basis]. Klinische Jahrbuch, 6, 299-326.

Ehrlich, P. (1900). On immunity with special reference to cell life. Proceedings Of The Royal Society Of London, 66(424-433), 424-448.
DOI: 10.1098/rspl.1899.0121

Ehrlich P. (1909) Über den jetzigen stand der karzinomforschung [Carcinoma research stood above the current one]. Ned Tijdschr Geneeskd; 5, 273-290.

Ellison, L. F., De, P., Mery, L. S., & Grundy, P. E. (2009). Canadian cancer statistics at a GLANCE: Cancer in children. Canadian Medical Association Journal, 180(4), 422-424. DOI: 10.1503/cmaj.081155

Eno, MS, PA-C, J. (2017). Immunotherapy Through the Years. Journal of the Advanced Practitioner in Oncology, 8(7). DOI: 10.6004/jadpro.2017.8.7.8

Fehleisen, F. (1882). Ueber die Züchtung der Erysipelkokken auf künstlichem Nährboden und ihre Uebertragbarkeit auf den Menschen [On the cultivation of the erysipelas on artificial culture medium and their transferability to humans]. Deutsche Medizinische Wochenschrift, 8(41), 553-554. DOI: 10.1055/s-0029-1196806

Farkona, S., Diamandis, E. P., & Blasutig, I. M. (2016). Cancer immunotherapy: The beginning of the end of cancer? BMC Medicine, 14(1). DOI: 10.1186/s12916-016-0623-5

Fong, A., Lafaro, K., Ituarte, P., & Fong, Y. (2021). Association of Living in Urban Food Deserts with Mortality from Breast and Colorectal Cancer. Annals of Surgical Oncology, 28(3), 1311–1319. DOI: 10.1245/s10434-020-09049-6

Forbes, L., Durocher-Allen, L.D., Vu, K., Gallo-Hershberg, D., Pardhan, A., Kennedy, K., Newton, J., Pitre, L., & Root, D. (2019). Regional models of care for systemic treatment: standards for the organization and delivery of systemic treatment. Toronto (ON): Ontario Cancer Care, 12-10.

Gajewski, T. F., Schreiber, H., & Fu, Y.-X. (2013). Innate and adaptive immune cells in the tumour microenvironment. Nature Immunology, 14(10), 1014–1022. DOI: 10.1038/ni.2703

Gasser, S., Orsulic, S., Brown, E. J., & Raulet, D. H. (2005). The DNA damage pathway regulates innate immune system ligands of the NKG2D receptor. Nature, 436(7054), 1186–1190. DOI: 10.1038/nature03884

Gilboa, E. (2004). The promise of cancer vaccines. Nature Reviews Cancer, 4(5), 401–411. DOI: 10.1038/nrc1359

Gresser, I., & Bourali, C. (1969). Exogenous Interferon and Inducers of Interferon in the Treatment of Balb/c Mice inoculated with RC19 Tumour Cells. Nature, 223(5208), 844–845. DOI: 10.1038/223844a0

Gupta, S. K., Jaitly, T., Schmitz, U., Schuler, G., Wolkenhauer, O., & Vera, J. (2015). Personalized cancer immunotherapy using Systems Medicine approaches. Briefings in Bioinformatics, 17(3), 453–467.
DOI: 10.1093/bib/bbv046

Hamilton, G., & Rath, B. (2019). Immunotherapy for small cell lung cancer: mechanisms of resistance. Expert Opinion on Biological Therapy, 19(5), 423–432.
DOI: 10.1080/14712598.2019.1592155

Harel, M., Ortenberg, R., Varanasi, S. K., Mangalhara, K. C., Mardamshina, M., Markovits, E., … Geiger, T. (2019). Proteomics of Melanoma Response to Immunotherapy Reveals Mitochondrial Dependence. Cell, 179(1), 236–250.
DOI: 10.1016/j.cell.2019.08.012

Hargadon, K.M., Johnson, C.E., & Williams, C.J. (2018). Immune checkpoint blockade therapy for cancer: An overview of FDA-approved immune checkpoint inhibitors. International Immunopharmacology, 62, 29-39.
DOI: 10.1016/j.intimp.2018.06.001

Helpman, L., Pond, G., Elit, L., & Seow, H. (2020). Social determinants of health in uterine cancer patients in Ontario: Association with disease presentation and outcomes. Gynecologic Oncology, 159(1), 66–66.
DOI: 10.1016/j.ygyno.2020.06.136

Holdcroft A. (2007). Gender bias in research: how does it affect evidence-based medicine?. Journal of the Royal Society of Medicine, 100(1), 2–3.
DOI: 10.1177/014107680710000102

Hoption Cann, S. A., van Netten, J. P., & van Netten, C. (2003). Dr William Coley and tumour regression: a place in history or in the future. Postgraduate medical journal, 79(938), 672–680.

How Immunotherapy Is Used to Treat Cancer.
(n.d.). Retrieved May 6, 2021, from https://www.cancer.org/treatment/treatments-and-side-effects/treatment-types/immunotherapy/what-is-immunotherapy.html

How Radiation Therapy Is Used to Treat Cancer. (n.d.). Retrieved May 6, 2021, from https://www.cancer.org/treatment/treatments-and-side-effects/treatment-types/radiation/basics.html

Huang, W., Chen, J.-J., Xing, R., & Zeng, Y.-Can. (2021). Combination Therapy: Future Directions of Immunotherapy in Small Cell Lung Cancer, 14(1).
DOI: 10.1016/j.tranon.2020.100889

Hutch, F. (2016, March 18). 6 questions in cancer immunotherapy. Fred Hutch. https://www.fredhutch.org/en/news/center-news/2016/03/6-questions-cancer-immunotherapy.html.

Iams, W. T., Shiuan, E., Meador, C. B., Roth, M., Bordeaux, J., Vaupel, C., Boyd, K.L., Summitt, I.B., Wang, L.L., Schneider, J.T., Warner, J.L., & Lovly, C. M. (2019). Improved Prognosis And Increased tumour-Infiltrating Lymphocytes in Patients Who Have SCLC With Neurologic Paraneoplastic Syndromes. Journal of Thoracic Oncology, 14(11), 1970–1981. DOI: 10.1016/j.jtho.2019.05.042

Igarashi, Y. & Sasada, T. (2020). Cancer vaccines: Toward the next breakthrough in cancer immunotherapy. Journal of Immunology Research. DOI: 10.1155/2020/5825401

Isaacs, A., & Lindenmann, J. (1957). Virus interference. I. The interferon. Proceedings of the Royal Society of London. Series B-Biological Sciences, 147(927), 258-267. DOI: 10.1098/rspb.1957.0048

Ivanovski, T., & Miralles, F. (2019). Lambert-Eaton Myasthenic syndrome: early diagnosis is key. Degenerative Neurological and Neuromuscular Disease, Volume 9, 27–37. DOI: 10.2147/dnnd.s192588

Ivers, L., & Ivers, L. (2015). Food Insecurity and Public Health. CRC Press.https://www-taylorfrancis-com.myaccess.library.utoronto.ca/chapters/mono/10.1201/b18451-11/food-insecurity-noncommunicable-diseases-among-poorest-louise-ivers?context=ubx&refId=3987b7e7-cecf-4c46-88fc-d5e9a7bb2e99

Jenkins, R., Barbie, D., & Flaherty, K. (2018). Mechanisms of resistance to immune checkpoint inhibitors. British Journal of Cancer, 118, 9-16. DOI: 10.1038/bjc.2017.434

Jiang, J., Ding, Y., Wu, M., Chen, Y., Lyu, X., Lu, J., Wang, H., & Teng, L. (2020). Integrated genomic analysis identifies a genetic mutation model predicting response to immune checkpoint inhibitors in melanoma. Cancer Medicine, 9(22), 8498–8518. DOI: 10.1002/cam4.3481

Johansson, H., Andersson, R., Bauden, M., Hammes, S., Holdenrieder, S., & Ansari, D. (2016). Immune checkpoint therapy for pancreatic cancer. World journal of gastroenterology, 22(43), 9457-9476. DOI: 10.3748/wjg.v22.i43.9457

June, C. H. (2007). Adoptive T cell therapy for cancer in the clinic. In Journal of Clinical Investigation (Vol. 117, Issue 6, pp. 1466–1476). American Society for Clinical Investigation. DOI: 10.1172/JCI32446

June, C. H., & Sadelain, M. (2018). Chimeric Antigen Receptor Therapy. New England Journal of Medicine, 379(1), 64–73. DOI: 10.1056/NEJMra1706169

Khair, D.O., Bax, H.J., Mele, S., Crescioli, S., Pellizzari, G., Khiabany, A., Nakamura, M., Harris, R.J., French, E., Hoffmann, R.M., Williams, I.P., Cheung, A., Thair, B., Beales,

C.T., Tour, E., Signell, A.W., Tasnova, N.L., Spicer, J.F., Josephs, D.H., ... Karagiannis, S.N. (2019). Combining Immune Checkpoint Inhibitors: Established and Emerging Targets and Strategies to Improve Outcomes in Melanoma. Frontiers in Immunology, 19. DOI: 10.3389/fimmu.2019.00453

Kienle G. S. (2012). Fever in Cancer Treatment: Coley's Therapy and Epidemiologic Observations. Global advances in health and medicine, 1(1), 92–100. DOI: 10.7453/gahmj.2012.1.1.016

Koury, J., Lucero, M., Cato, C., Chang, L., Geiger, J., Henry, D., ... Tran, A. (2018). Immunotherapies: Exploiting the Immune System for Cancer Treatment. Journal of Immunology Research, 2018, 1–16. DOI: 10.1155/2018/9585614

Kruger, S., Ilmer, M., Kobold, S., Cadilha, B. L., Endres, S., Ormanns, S. von Bergwelt-Baildon, M. (2019). Advances in cancer immunotherapy 2019 – latest trends. Journal of Experimental and Clinical Cancer Research, 38(1). DOI: 10.1186/s13046-019-1266-0

Lake, J. P., Pierce, C. W., & Kennedy, J. D. (1991). T Cell receptor expression by T cells that mature extrathymically in nude mice. Cellular Immunology, 135(1), 259–265. DOI: 10.1016/0008-8749(91)90270-l

Larbi, A., & Fulop, T. (2014). From "truly naïve" to "exhausted senescent" T cells: When markers predict functionality. In Cytometry Part A (Vol. 85, Issue 1, pp. 25–35). John Wiley & Sons, Ltd. DOI: 10.1002/cyto.a.22351

Lee, H. J., Kim, Y. A., Sim, C. K., Heo, S. H., Song, I. H., Park, H. S., Park, S. Y., Bang, W. S., Park, I. A., Lee, M., Lee, J. H., Cho, Y. S., Chang, S., Jung, J., Kim, J., Lee, S. B., Kim, S. Y., Lee, M. S., & Gong, G. (2017). Expansion of tumour-infiltrating lymphocytes and their potential for application as adoptive cell transfer therapy in human breast cancer. Oncotarget, 8(69), 113345–113359. DOI: 10.18632/oncotarget.23007

Lee, S., & Margolin, K. (2012). tumour-infiltrating lymphocytes in melanoma. Current Oncology Reports, 14(5), 468–474. DOI: 10.1007/s11912-012-0257-5

Lee, S. (n.d.). Cancer statistics at a glance. https://action.cancer.ca/en/research/cancer-statistics/cancer-statistics-at-a-glance

Lesterhuis, W. J., Punt, C. J. A., Hato, S. V., Eleveld-Trancikova, D., Jansen, B. J. H., Nierkens, S., Schreibelt, G., de Boer, A., Van Herpen, C.M., Kaanders, J.H., van Krieken, J.H., & de Vries, I. J. (2011). Platinum-based drugs disrupt STAT6-mediated suppression of immune responses against cancer in humans and mice. Journal of Clinical Investigation, 121(8), 3100–3108. DOI: 10.1172/jci43656

Maher, J., Brentjens, R. J., Gunset, G., Rivière, I., & Sadelain, M. (2002). Human T-lymphocyte cytotoxicity and proliferation directed by a single chimeric TCRζ/CD28 receptor. Nature biotechnology, 20(1), 70-75.
DOI: 10.1038/nbt0102-70

Make it Safe. (2020, May 27). Human Rights Watch. https://www.hrw.org/report/2016/06/07/make-it-safe/canadas-obligation-end-first-nations-water-crisis

Majzner, R. G., & Mackall, C. L. (2018). Tumour antigen escape from car t-cell therapy. In Cancer Discovery (Vol. 8, Issue 10, pp. 1219–1226). American Association for Cancer Research Inc.
DOI: 10.1158/2159-8290.CD-18-0442

Marmot, M. (2018). Health equity, cancer, and social determinants of health. The Lancet Global Health, 6, S29–S29.
DOI: 10.1016/S2214-109X(18)30098-6

Martins, F., Sofiya, L., Sykiotis, G.P. Lamine, F., Maillard, M., Fraga, M., Shabafrouz, K., Ribi, C., Cairoli, A., Guex-Crosier, Y., Kuntzer, T., Michielin, O., Peters, S., Coukos, G., Spertini, F., Thompson, J.A., & Obeid, M. (2019). Adverse effects of immune-checkpoint inhibitors: epidemiology, management and surveillance. Nature Reviews Clinical Oncology, 16, 563-580.
DOI: 10.1038/s41571-019-0218-0

Martuza, R. L., Malick, A., Markert, J. M., Ruffner, K. L., & Coen, D. M. (1991). Experimental therapy of human glioma by means of a genetically engineered virus mutant. Science, 252(5007), 854-856.
DOI: 10.1126/science.1851332

Maserejian, N. N., Link, C. L., Lutfey, K. L., Marceau, L. D., & McKinlay, J. B. (2009). Disparities in physicians' interpretations of heart disease symptoms by patient gender: results of a video vignette factorial experiment. Journal of women's health (2002), 18(10), 1661–1667.
DOI: 10.1089/jwh.2008.1007

Mayer, A. T., Natarajan, A., Gordon, S. R., Maute, R. L., McCracken, M. N., Ring, A. M., Weissman, I. L., & Gambhir, S. S. (2016). Practical Immuno-PET Radiotracer Design Considerations for Human Immune Checkpoint Imaging. Journal of Nuclear Medicine, 58(4), 538–546.
DOI: 10.2967/jnumed.116.177659

McCarthy E. F. (2006). The toxins of William B. Coley and the treatment of bone and soft-tissue sarcomas. The Iowa orthopedic journal, 26, 154–158.
DOI: 10.2147%2FITT.S163924

Miao, L., Zhang, Y. & Huang, L. (2021). mRNA vaccine for cancer immunotherapy. Molecular Cancer.
DOI: 10.1186/s12943-021-01335-5

Mohanty, R., Chowdhury, C. R., Arega, S., Sen, P., Ganguly, P., & Ganguly, N. (2019). CAR T cell therapy: A new era for cancer treatment (Review). In Oncology Reports (Vol. 42, Issue 6, pp. 2183–2195). Spandidos Publications. DOI: 10.3892/or.2019.7335

Morales, A., Eidinger, D., & Bruce, A. W. (1976). Intracavitary Bacillus Calmette-Guerin in the treatment of superficial bladder tumours. The Journal of urology, 167(2), 891-894. Morgan, D. A., Ruscetti, F. W., & Gallo, R. (1976). Selective in vitro growth of T lymphocytes from normal human bone marrows. Science, 193(4257), 1007-1008. DOI: 10.1126/science.181845

Murciano-Goroff, Y. R., Warner, A. B., & Wolchok, J. D. (2020). The future of cancer immunotherapy: microenvironment-targeting combinations. Cell Research, 30(6), 507–519. DOI: 10.1038/s41422-020-0337-2

Murdoch, B. (2020). The legal and policy considerations of transplanting pediatric thymus regulatory T cells as an immunotherapy in Canada. Medical Law International, 20(3), 201-210. DOI: 10.1177/0968533220963157

Nash, A. (2015). The Consuming Geographies of Food: Diet, Food Deserts and Obesity by Hillary J. Shaw, Routledge, London and New York, 2014, (ISBN 978-0415818704). The Canadian Geographer, 59(3), e83–e83. DOI: 10.1111/cag.12213

Nelson, B. (2017). Customizing cancer immunotherapies to match the intrinsic tumour microenvironment. British Columbia Cancer Agency Precision Medicine Retreat. August 9, 2017.

Nishimura, H., Nose, M., Hiai, H., Minato, N., & Honjo, T. (1999). Development of lupus-like autoimmune diseases by disruption of the PD-1 gene encoding an ITIM motif-carrying immunoreceptor. Immunity, 11(2), 141-151. DOI: 10.1016/S1074-7613(00)80089-8

Nishino, M., Hatabu, H., & Hodi, F. S. (2019). Imaging of Cancer Immunotherapy: Current Approaches and Future Directions. Radiology, 290(1), 9–22. DOI: 10.1148/radiol.2018181349

Oiseth, S., & Aziz, M. (2017). Cancer immunotherapy: a brief review of the history, possibilities, and challenges ahead. Journal Of Cancer Metastasis And Treatment, 3(10), 250. DOI: 10.20517/2394-4722.2017.41

Old, L. J., Clarke, D. A., & Benacerraf, B. (1959). Effect of Bacillus Calmette-Guérin Infection on Transplanted Tumours in the Mouse. Nature, 184(4682), 291–292. DOI: 10.1038/184291a0

Patt, D., Gordan, L., Diaz, M., Okon, T., Grady, L., Harmison, M., Markward, N., Sullivan, M., Peng, J., & Zhou, A. (2020). Impact of COVID-19 on Cancer Care: How the Pandemic Is Delaying Cancer Diagnosis and Treatment for American Seniors. JCO clinical cancer informatics, 4, 1059–1071.
DOI: 10.1200/CCI.20.00134

Parish, C. (2003). Cancer immunotherapy: The past, the present and the future. Immunology & Cell Biology, 81(2), 106-113.
DOI:10.1046/j.0818-9641.2003.01151.x

Pearl, R. (1929). Cancer and tuberculosis. American Journal of Hygiene, 9, 97-159.

Pfannenstiel, L. W., McNeilly, C., Xiang, C., Kang, K., Diaz-Montero, C. M., Yu, J. S., & Gastman, B. R. (2018). Combination PD-1 blockade and irradiation of brain metastasis induce an effective abscopal effect in melanoma. OncoImmunology, 8(1).
DOI: 10.1080/2162402x.2018.1507669

Puglisi, M., Dolly, S., Faria, A., Myerson, J. S., Popat, S., & O'Brien, M. E. (2010). Treatment options for small cell lung cancer – do we have more choice? British Journal of Cancer, 102(4), 629–638.
DOI: 10.1038/sj.bjc.6605527

Radvanyi, L. G., Bernatchez, C., Zhang, M., Fox, P. S., Miller, P., Chacon, J., Wu, R., Lizee, G., Mahoney, S., Alvarado, G., Glass, M., Johnson, V. E., McMannis, J. D., Shpall, E., Prieto, V., Papadopoulos, N., Kim, K., Homsi, J., Bedikian, A., ... Hwu, P. (2012). Specific lymphocyte subsets predict response to adoptive cell therapy using expanded autologous tumour-infiltrating lymphocytes in metastatic melanoma patients. Clinical Cancer Research, 18(24), 6758–6770.
DOI: 10.1158/1078-0432.CCR-12-1177

Ramos, C. A., & Dotti, G. (2011). Chimeric antigen receptor (CAR)-engineered lymphocytes for cancer therapy. In Expert Opinion on Biological Therapy (Vol. 11, Issue 7, pp. 855–873). Taylor & Francis.
DOI: 10.1517/14712598.2011.573476

Reck, M., Vicente, D., Ciuleanu, T., Gettinger, S., Peters, S., Horn, L., Audigier-Valette, C., Pardo, N., Juan-Vidal, O., Cheng, Y., Zhang, H., & Spigel, D. R. (2018). Efficacy and safety of nivolumab (Nivo) monotherapy versus chemotherapy (chemo) in recurrent small cell lung cancer (SCLC): Results from CheckMate 331. Annals of Oncology, 29, x43.
DOI: 10.1093/annonc/mdy511.004

Rohaan, M. W., van den Berg, J. H., Kvistborg, P., & Haanen, J. B. A. G. (2018). Adoptive transfer of tumour-infiltrating lymphocytes in melanoma: A viable treatment option 11 Medical and Health Sciences 1107 Immunology 11 Medical and Health Sciences 1112 Oncology and Carcinogenesis. In Journal for ImmunoTherapy of Cancer (Vol. 6, Issue 1, p. 102). BioMed Central Ltd.
DOI: 10.1186/s40425-018-0391-1

Rosenberg, S. A., Yang, J. C., Sherry, R. M., Kammula, U. S., Hughes, M. S., Phan, G. Q., Citrin, D. E., Restifo, N. P., Robbins, P. F., Wunderlich, J. R., Morton, K. E., Laurencot, C. M., Steinberg, S. M., White, D. E., & Dudley, M. E. (2011). Durable complete responses in heavily pretreated patients with metastatic melanoma using T-cell transfer immuno-therapy. Clinical Cancer Research, 17(13), 4550–4557.
DOI: 10.1158/1078-0432.CCR-11-0116

Ruan, H., Bu, L., Hu, Q., Cheng, H., Lu, W., & Gu, Z. (2019). Strategies of Combination Drug Delivery for Immune Checkpoint Blockades. Advanced Healthcare Materials, 8(4), e1801099.
DOI: 10.1002/adhm.201801099.

Salim, S. K., Xu, J., Wong, N., Venugopal, C., Hope, K. J., & Singh, S. K. (2020). Assess-ing the Safety of a Cell-Based Immunotherapy for Brain Cancers Using a Humanized Model of Hematopoiesis. STAR protocols, 1(3), 100124.
DOI: 10.1016/j.xpro.2020.100124

Schmitt, T. M., Ragnarsson, G. B., & Greenberg, P. D. (2009). T cell receptor gene ther-apy for cancer. In Human Gene Therapy (Vol. 20, Issue 11, pp. 1240–1248). Mary Ann Liebert, Inc. 140 Huguenot Street, 3rd Floor New Rochelle, NY 10801 USA
DOI: 10.1089/hum.2009.146

Schuster, M., Nechansky, A., & Kircheis, R. (2006). Cancer immunotherapy, Biotech-nology Journal, 1(2), 138-147.
DOI: 10.1002/biot.200500044

Schwartz, R. S. (1997). Book Review A Commotion in the Blood: Life, death, and the immune system By Stephen S. Hall. 544 pp. New York, Henry Holt, 1997. $30. 0-8050-3796-9. New England Journal of Medicine, 337(16), 1178–1179.
DOI: 10.1056/nejm199710163371621

Sen, T., Rodriguez, B. L., Chen, L., Corte, C. M., Morikawa, N., Fujimoto, J., ... Byers, L. A. (2019). Targeting DNA Damage Response Promotes Antitumour Immunity through STING-Mediated T-cell Activation in Small Cell Lung Cancer. Cancer Discovery, 9(5), 646–661.
DOI: 10.1158/2159-8290.cd-18-1020

Sharma, P., Siddiqui, B.A., Anandhan, S., Yadav, S.S., Subudhi, S.K., Gao, J., Goswami, S., & Allison, J.P. (2021). The Next Decade of Immune Checkpoint Therapy. Cancer Discovery, 11(4), 838-857.
DOI: 10.1158/2159-8290.CD-20-1680.

Shaver's, V., Brown, M. Racial and Ethnic Disparities in the Receipt of Cancer Treat-ment, JNCI: Journal of the National Cancer Institute, Volume 94, Issue 5, 6 March 2002, Pages 334–357,
DOI: 10.1093/jnci/94.5.334

Shibata, H., Zhou, L., Xu, N., Egloff, A.M. & Uppaluri, R. (2020). Personalized cancer vaccination in head and neck cancer. Cancer Science, 112, 978-988.
DOI: 10.1111/cas.14784

Slingluff, C. L., Jr. (2019). Building on the promise of a cancer vaccine for solid tumours. Clinical Cancer Research, 26(3), 529-531.
DOI: 10.1158/1078-0432.CCR-19-3206

Solinas, C., Gombos, A., Latifyan, S., Piccart-Gebhart, M., Kok, M., & Buisseret, L. (2017). Targeting immune checkpoints in breast cancer: an update of early results. Science Direct, 2(5), e000255.
DOI: 10.1136/esmoopen-2017-000255.

Stutman, O. (1974). Tumour development after 3-methylcholanthrene in immunologically deficient athymic-nude mice. Science, 183(4124), 534-536.
DOI: 10.1126/science.183.4124.534

Tagliaferri, L., Garganese, G., D'Aviero, A., Lancellotta, V., Fragomeni, S.M., Fionda, B., Casà, C., Gui, B., Perotti, G., Gentileschi, S., & Inzani, F. (2020). Multidisciplinary personalized approach in the management of vulvar cancer–the Vul. Can Team experience. International Journal of Gynecologic Cancer, 30(7).
DOI: 10.1136/ijgc-2020-001465

Thomas, L., & Lawrence, H. S. (1959). Cellular and Humoral Aspects of the Hypersensitive States: A Symposium at the New York Academy of Medicine. Journal of the American Medical Association, 170(7), 883.
DOI: 10.1001/jama.1959.03010070123025

Vahabi, M., Lofters, A., Kumar, M., & Glazier, R. (2016). Breast cancer screening disparities among immigrant women by world region of origin: a population-based study in Ontario, Canada. Cancer Medicine (Malden, MA), 5(7), 1670–1686.
DOI: 10.1002/cam4.700

Verma, V., Haque, W., Cushman, T. R., Lin, C., Simone, C. B., 2nd, Chang, J. Y., McClelland, S., 3rd, & Welsh, J. W. (2019). Racial and Insurance-related Disparities in Delivery of Immunotherapy-type Compounds in the United States. Journal of immunotherapy (Hagerstown, Md.: 1997), 42(2), 55–64.
DOI: 10.1097/CJI.0000000000000253

Vernon L. F. (2018). William Bradley Coley, MD, and the phenomenon of spontaneous regression. ImmunoTargets and therapy, 7, 29–34.
DOI: 10.2147/ITT.S163924

Vinay, D. S., Ryan, E. P., Pawelec, G., Talib, W. H., Stagg, J., Elkord, E., Lichtor, T., Decker, W. K., Whelan, R. L., Kumara, H. M. C. S., Signori, E., Honoki, K., Georgakilas, A. G., Amin, A., Helferich, W. G., Boosani, C. S., Guha, G., Ciriolo, M. R., Chen, S., ... Kwon, B. S. (2015). Immune evasion in cancer: Mechanistic basis and therapeutic strategies.

Seminars in Cancer Biology, 35, S185–S198.
DOI: 10.1016/j.semcancer.2015.03.004

Haque, W., Verma, V., Butler, E. B., & Teh, B. S. (2019). Racial and Socioeconomic Disparities in the Delivery of Immunotherapy for Metastatic Melanoma in the United States. Journal of immunotherapy (Hagerstown, Md.: 1997), 42(6), 228–235.
DOI: 10.1097/CJI.0000000000000264

Wang, X.-Y., & Fisher, P. B. (2019). Preface. Advances in Cancer Research, xiii-xv.
DOI: 10.1016/s0065-230x(19)30049-1

Webster, R. (2014). The immune checkpoint inhibitors: where are we now?. Nature Reviews Drug Discovery, 13, 883–884.
DOI: 10.1038/nrd4476

Weichselbaum, R. R., Liang, H., Deng, L., & Fu, Y.-X. (2017). Radiotherapy and immunotherapy: a beneficial liaison? Nature Reviews Clinical Oncology, 14(6), 365–379.
DOI: 10.1038/nrclinonc.2016.211

What causes cancer? - Canadian Cancer Society. (n.d.). Retrieved from https://www.cancer.ca/en/cancer-information/cancer-101/what-causes-cancer/?region=on

What Is Cancer? - National Cancer Institute (nciglobal,ncienterprise). (2007, September 17). [CgvArticle]. https://www.cancer.gov/about-cancer/understanding/what-is-cancer

Why People with Cancer Are More Likely to Get Infections. (n.d.). Retrieved May 6, 2021, from https://www.cancer.org/treatment/treatments-and-side-effects/physical-side-effects/low-blood-counts/infections/why-people-with-cancer-are-at-risk.html

William B. Coley Award. (2020). Cancer Research Institute. https://www.cancerresearch.org/about-cri/awards-honors/william-b-coley-award

Wu, R., Forget, M. A., Chacon, J., Bernatchez, C., Haymaker, C., Chen, J. Q., Hwu, P., & Radvanyi, L. G. (2012). Adoptive T-cell therapy using autologous tumour-infiltrating lymphocytes for metastatic melanoma: Current status and future outlook. In Cancer Journal (Vol. 18, Issue 2, pp. 160–175). NIH Public Access.
DOI: 10.1097/PPO.0b013e31824d4465

Xu, F., Jin, T., Zhu, Y., & Dai, C. (2018). Immune checkpoint therapy in liver cancer. Journal of Experimental and Clinical Cancer Research, 110(37).
DOI: 10.1186/s13046-018-0777-4

Xu, Z., Zeng, S., Gong, Z. & Yan, Y. (2020). Exome-based immunotherapy: a promising approach for cancer treatment. Molecular Cancer.
DOI: 10.1186/s12943-020-01278-3

Zavitz, C. "Immunology 1: Innate Immunity". Human Physiology and Anatomy II 2FF3. February 2021. McMaster University. Class Lecture

Zhang, H., & Chen, J. (2018). Current status and future directions of cancer immuno-therapy. Journal of Cancer, 9(10), 1773–1781.
DOI: 10.7150/jca.24577

Zhang, R., Liu, T., Tsuchiya, N., Mashima, H., Kobayashi, T., Nakatsura, T., Uemura, Y. (2021). Induced pluripotent stem cell-derived, genetically engineered myeloid cells as unlimited cell sources for dendritic cell-related cancer immunotherapy. Journal of Immunology and Regenerative Medicine, 12, 100042.
DOI: 10.1016/j.regen.2021.100042

Zhou, L., Lu, L., Wicha, M. S., Chang, A. E., Xia, J., Ren, X. & Li, Q. (2015). The promise of cancer stem cell vaccine. Human Vaccines & Immunotherapeutics, 11(12), 2796-2799.
DOI: 10.1080/21645515.2015.1083661

www.ingramcontent.com/pod-product-compliance
Lightning Source LLC
Chambersburg PA
CBHW030852270326
41928CB00008B/1342